Leadership

Guest Editors

PATRICIA S. YODER-WISE, RN, EdD, NEA-BC, ANEF, FAAN
KARREN KOWALSKI, PhD, RN, NEA-BC, FAAN

NURSING CLINICS
OF NORTH AMERICA

www.nursing.theclinics.com

Consulting Editor
SUZANNE S. PREVOST, RN, PhD, COI

March 2010 • Volume 45 • Number 1

SAUNDERS an imprint of ELSEVIER, Inc.

W.B. SAUNDERS COMPANY
A Division of Elsevier Inc.

1600 John F. Kennedy Blvd., Suite 1800 • Philadelphia, PA 19103-2899

http://www.theclinics.com

NURSING CLINICS OF NORTH AMERICA Volume 45, Number 1
March 2010 ISSN 0029-6465, ISBN-13: 978-1-4377-1890-4

Editor: Katie Hartner
Developmental Editor: Donald Mumford

Nursing Clinics of North America (ISSN 0029-6465) is published quarterly by Elsevier Inc., 360 Park Avenue South, New York, NY 10010-1710. Months of issue are March, June, September, and December. Periodicals postage paid at New York, NY and additional mailing offices. Subscription price per year is, $133.00 (US individuals), $306.00 (US institutions), $228.00 (international individuals), $374.00 (international institutions), $184.00 (Canadian individuals), $374.00 (Canadian institutions), $70.00 (US students), and $115.00 (international students). To receive student/resident rate, orders must be accompanied by name of affiliated institution, date of term, and the signature of program/residency coordinator on institution letterhead. Orders will be billed at individual rate until proof of status is received. Foreign air speed delivery is included in all *Clinics* subscription prices. All prices are subject to change without notice. **POSTMASTER:** Send address changes to *Nursing Clinics*, Elsevier Health Sciences Division, Subscription Customer Service, 3251 Riverport Lane, Maryland Heights, MO 63043. **Customer Service: Telephone: 1-800-654-2452** (U.S. and Canada); **1-314-447-8871 (outside U.S. and Canada). Fax: 1-314-447-8029. E-mail: journalscustomerservice-usa@elsevier.com** (for print support) and **journalsonlinesupport-usa@elsevier.com** (for online support).

Nursing Clinics of North America is covered in *EMBASE/Excerpta Medica, MEDLINE/PubMed (Index Medicus), Social Sciences Citation Index, Current Contents, ASCA, Cumulative Index to Nursing, RNdex Top 100,* and Allied Health Literature and International Nursing Index (INI).

Printed and bound by CPI Group (UK) Ltd, Croydon, CR0 4YY

Transferred to Digital Print 2011

Contributors

CONSULTING EDITOR

SUZANNE S. PREVOST, PhD, RN, COI
Associate Dean, Practice and Community Engagement, University of Kentucky, Lexington, Kentucky

GUEST EDITORS

PATRICIA S. YODER-WISE, RN, EdD, NEA-BC, ANEF, FAAN
President, The Wise Group, Lubbock, Texas

KARREN KOWALSKI, PhD, RN, NEA-BC, FAAN
Grant/Project Director, Colorado Center for Nursing Excellence, Denver, Colorado; Professor, Anita Thigpen Perry School of Nursing, Texas Tech University, Lubbock, Texas

AUTHORS

JOYCE BATCHELLER, MSN, RN, NEA-BC, FAAN
Senior Vice President, System Chief Nursing Officer, Seton Family of Hospitals, Austin, Texas

ELAINE COHEN, RN, EdD, FAAN
Associate Chief of Nursing, QI, James A. Haley Veterans' Hospital, Tampa, Florida

ROBERT L. DENT, DNP, MBA, RN, NEA-BC, FACHE
Midland Memorial Hospital, Midland, Texas

KATHY DOUGLAS, MHA, RN
President, Institute for Staffing Excellence & Innovation, Sedona, Arizona

MARYANN F. FRALIC, RN, DrPH, FAAN
Professor, Johns Hopkins University School of Nursing, Baltimore, Maryland; Executive Advisor, The Nursing Executive Center of the Advisory Board Company, Washington, DC

MARGO A. KARSTEN, RN, BSN, MSN, PhD
Faculty Member, University of Colorado, Windsor, Colorado

KARLENE KERFOOT, PhD, RN, NEA-BC, FAAN
Vice President and Chief Clinical Officer, Aurora Health Care, Milwaukee, Wisconsin

KATHY MALLOCH, PhD, MBA, RN, FAAN
President, Kathy Malloch Leadership Systems, Glendale; Clinical Professor, Arizona State University, College of Nursing and Health Innovation, Phoenix, Arizona; Clinical Consultant, API Healthcare, Hartford, Wisconsin

CAROL A. MANNAHAN, EdD, RN, NEA-BC
Professor Emeritus, University of Oklahoma College of Nursing, Oklahoma City, Oklahoma

ERIN K. MEREDITH, ARNP-BC, PCCN
Assistant Chief of Nursing, QI/Magnet Program Director, James A. Haley Veterans' Hospital, Tampa, Florida

LUCILLE V. RAIA, RN, MS, ARNP-BC, NEA-BC
Associate Chief of Nursing, Nursing Education, James A. Haley Veterans' Hospital, Tampa, Florida

Contents

The industrial age command and control leadership style and supporting infrastructure are ineffective in meeting the challenges of the increased availability and sharing of information, the media used for knowledge transfer, the changing range and types of relationships between individuals, and the time required to transfer and share information. What has not changed is the need for effective personal relationships in the evaluation and selection of new technologies; human to human sensitivity, acknowledgment, and respect for the patient care experience. As individuals embrace these new technologies, the essence of the innovation leader emerges to purposefully guide, assess, integrate, and synthesize technology into the human work of patient care. Building organizational infrastructures with openness for technology and innovations to enhance effective patient care relationships now requires an innovation skill set that understands and integrates human needs with the best of technology. In this article a brief description of innovation leadership is presented as the backdrop for change along with 4 significant changes in work processes that have irreversibly altered health care work, the trimodal organizational structure to accommodate operations, innovation, and transition between the 2, and finally, individual and team behaviors that emphasize the work of innovation.

The complexity of care, increased cost pressures, nursing shortage, competition for experienced nurses, and focus on "never events" are some of the challenges faced by chief nursing officers (CNOs). The CNO is the executive leader for the largest and most influential group of professionals in most health care organizations. He or she can provide transformational changes that are needed to address issues such as those cited in the opening sentence. For this reason an in-depth literature review was performed to summarize key findings and factors that contribute to the high CNO turnover. The results of this review can be used as the basis for planning strategies to assist new and current CNOs in their development to reverse this turnover trend.

How does today's nurse executive function effectively within an incredibly complex health care environment? Does it require different skills, new

competencies, new behaviors? Can nurse executives, irrespective of setting, who have always been successful in the past, move forward with the
same strategic and operational behaviors? Is there "new work" associated
with a new context for executive practice? To answer these questions, this
article considers key contemporary issues.

Organizations are transitioning from a management industrial era to a humanistic era. This transition will require a different set of leadership competencies. Competencies that reflect relationships, connections with
employees, and having the skill to unleash the human capability at all levels
of an organization are essential. Similar to when a sports team needs a different play book to be successful, leaders need a new play book. Coaches
within the sports team are the ones who assist players in learning how to
adapt to a different set of rules. They teach the players how to show up differently and how to implement different plays, with the overall goal of being
a successful team. New competencies are being required to reflect a humanistic approach to leadership. It is critical that organizations offer
coaching as an intervention to all levels of leadership. This actual case
study demonstrates that coaching not only assisted leaders in learning
a new way of leading but also improved overall organizational effectiveness. The results that have been accomplished through the use of implementing a 360-degree feedback system, with coaching, reaped overall
organization improvement.

The many benefits to hospitals throughout the world that achieved Magnet
designation is well documented. This status of recognition demands the
support of leadership during the Magnet journey. In 2008, the American
Nurses Credentialing Center (ANCC) announced a new model for the Magnet Recognition Program that translates the original 14 Forces of Magnetism into Five Model Components. Specifically, this new model includes
sources of evidence and empiric outcomes that by definition accentuates
transformational nursing leadership. The day-to-day impact of this change
places an even greater emphasis on demonstrated outcomes and innovation that may potentially transform nursing practice, quality and safety of
care, and the population served. This article provides tangible examples
and outcomes for reaching nursing excellence through leadership support
and engagement.

One of the first encounters many people have with a health care institution
occurs in the emergency department. If that area presents a poor picture
to patients and their families, the whole institution can be seen as negative.
How a tertiary care facility identified a way to improve the appropriate use
of the emergency dept is the focus of this article.

Nurses and physicians have a unique opportunity to work together to provide quality patient care. Although numerous studies have documented the value of effective nurse-physician communication on patient outcomes and on nurse and physician satisfaction, communication between many physicians and nurses continues to be poor. A variety of reasons for this disconnect have been identified, including differences in education, role expectations, gender, and approach to practice. Based on the principle that it is more important to understand than to be understood, application of a cultural competence model offers nurses the opportunity to better understand their physician colleagues. Because of the imperative to provide sensitive care to a diverse population, nurses are expected to assess cultural variations when planning care. That same skill can be applied to improving professional relationships with physicians. This article proposes application of a cultural competence model as a framework to assist nurses to better understand physicians with whom they work. With a focus on how culture affects one's world view, nurses will be encouraged to employ this cultural competence model in their interactions with physicians.

Embracing an inclusive leadership style is the foundation of building an approach to staffing that maximizes outcomes for patients, the workforce, and the organizations in which care is delivered. By engaging everyone involved and inviting participation, a structure of shared understanding is created, providing an environment that is positioned to achieve optimal results. Communityship offers a model for approaching leadership that is aligned with leveraging talent across an organization and developing a culture prepared to face the complex challenges of staffing and achieving new levels of performance that an evidence-based approach to staffing excellence can offer. A zero-defect health care system can be achieved by developing communityship.

FORTHCOMING ISSUES

RECENT ISSUES

THE CLINICS ARE NOW AVAILABLE ONLINE!

Access your subscription at:
www.theclinics.com

Preface

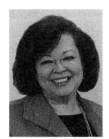

Karren Kowalski, PhD, RN, NEA-BC, FAAN
Guest Editor

Numerous issues face nursing leaders in today's challenging environments. We face concerns about patient safety and we note worrisome new data indicating that we have not made much headway in saving lives. Simultaneously, we try to reflect on what we have learned throughout our careers. Furthermore, we must also think about the future and what strategies we need to put in place to ready ourselves and our colleagues for what will evolve.

Nurse leaders must handle many challenges. These range from the simplest physician–nurse relationships, which inevitably turn out to be quite complex, to the demanding expectations stemming from Magnet's new outcomes. This story—the story of what it takes to be a nurse leader and how nurse leaders today come to grips with so many issues—may be told in many ways. This issue of *Nursing Clinics of North America* contains multiple views and reflections on the importance of the role of nurse leaders and their commitment to transforming nursing.

As we read these manuscripts, we were struck with big-picture issues. How is it possible for chief nursing officers to transform cultures when the literature suggests there is a high turnover rate in that position? How can we meet the Institute of Medicine's expectations for health profession competencies when we have yet to bridge the communication gap with physicians? What has our experience taught us and how can we apply these lessons to help us live up to the new outcomes expectations? We don't guarantee that you come away from this issue of *Nursing Clinics of North America* with all of the answers. We do think, however, that you will find practical and inspirational ideas to continue your journey toward excellence in leadership.

Karren Kowalski, PhD, RN, NEA-BC, FAAN
Colorado Center for Nursing Excellence
5290 East Yale Circle #102
Denver, CO 80222, USA
Anita Thigpen Perry School of Nursing
Texas Tech University, Lubbock, TX, USA

E-mail address:
Karren.kowalski@worldnet.att.net

Nurs Clin N Am 45 (2010) ix
doi:10.1016/j.cnur.2010.01.001   **nursing.theclinics.com**
0029-6465/10/$ – see front matter © 2010 Elsevier Inc. All rights reserved.

Innovation Leadership: New Perspectives for New Work

Kathy Malloch, PhD, MBA, RN, FAAN[a,b,c,*]

KEYWORDS

- Innovation • Leadership • Vulnerability • Courage
- Trimodal leadership

As the world moves more and more deeply into the digital information age, the rapid-fire introduction of new technologies has dramatically changed the landscape for health care organizations. The tension between the need for reliable operations and the never-ending demand for innovation is often overwhelming. The time and location of work continues to evolve daily. Communication is possible to any location at any time, information is transported electronically, and speedy processing is the norm. Work does not require the physical presence of individuals, does not wait for documents to be delivered by postal services, and has little regard for traditional patterns and modes of communication. Individuals can now create, transfer, and communicate information at any time, anywhere in the world. These changes have created significant challenges for traditional leaders.

The industrial age command and control leadership style and supporting infrastructure are ineffective in meeting the challenges of the increased availability and sharing of information, the media used for knowledge transfer, the changing range and types of relationships between individuals, and the time required to transfer and share information. The authority delineation guidelines of the organization's chart and the Monday through Friday work schedules have been almost eliminated with the advances in the information age.

What has not changed is the need for effective personal relationships in the evaluation and selection of new technologies; human to human sensitivity, acknowledgment, and respect for the patient care experience. As individuals embrace these new technologies, the essence of the innovation leader or Quantum Leader emerges to purposefully guide, assess, integrate, and synthesize technology into the human work of patient care.[1] Building organizational infrastructures with openness for

[a] Kathy Malloch Leadership Systems, Glendale, AZ 85308, USA
[b] Arizona State University, College of Nursing and Health Innovation, 500 North 3rd Street, Phoenix, AZ 85004-0698, USA
[c] API Healthcare, Hartford, WI, USA
* Corresponding author. 7116 West Behrend Drive, Glendale, AZ.
E-mail address: km@kathymalloch.com

Nurs Clin N Am 45 (2010) 1–9
doi:10.1016/j.cnur.2009.10.001   nursing.theclinics.com

technology and innovations to enhance effective patient care relationships now requires an innovation skill set that understands and integrates human needs with the best of technology—not the reverse, integrating technology into work processes that minimizes or eliminates human encounters. In this article a brief description of innovation leadership is presented as the backdrop for change along with 4 significant changes in work processes that have irreversibly altered health care work, the trimodal organizational structure to accommodate operations, innovation, and transition between the 2, and finally, individual and team behaviors that emphasize the work of innovation.

INNOVATION LEADERSHIP IS...

Innovation leadership is a relatively new concept that provides a futuristic lens for leaders in the revolutionary digital age which has now reached critical mass.[1] Innovation leadership is defined as *the process of creating the context for innovation to occur; creating and implementing the roles, decision-making structures, physical space, partnerships, networks, and equipment that support innovative thinking and testing.*[2]

This innovation leadership role is necessary to analyze and synthesize the impact of the dramatic changes in the organizational infrastructure and achieve sustainable organizational results. Four specific changes created by digital products and processes, including the location of work, the media to share work, the time available for work, and the communication networks for sharing are dramatically changing the organizational landscape.[3]

Work location. The location for work is no longer limited to a specific physical space. The availability of the Internet renders the location of work less important. Physical office space needs are quite different, with the ability to communicate and process work from remote locations. Less and less work is performed in traditional office spaces and conference rooms. Further, patient care is not limited to the simultaneous presence of a patient and caregiver in the same physical place; virtual care models are becoming more available.

Media for work. The sharing and transferring of work products has been accelerated with the use of digital transfer media. Anyone can publish content on the Internet for anyone with social networking (Web 2.0) technology. Work products are no longer limited to paper, pen, and file cabinets.

Time for work. Work now can be done immediately, at any time, in any place. Work is no longer restricted to a designated time span, namely office hours or designated shift length. The widespread availability of the Internet, shared files, and social networks makes time nearly irrelevant. Work now occurs at any time across the globe. Real-time communication resources have significantly decreased waiting time. Further, it is now possible to schedule time with multiple individuals in much less time. Individuals are no longer waiting for the mail to arrive; the mail (e-mail) is waiting for the individual to process.

Communication. The fourth change impacts organizational structures and authority lines. The organizational chart may indicate communication lines between hierarchal levels; however, the availability of electronic e-mails and social networks now eliminates those designated communication lines. Any individual can communicate with leaders at any time about any subject or issue. The availability of text messaging, instant messaging, and social networks have dramatically changed organizational work processes. At one time the CEO would learn about an issue at scheduled meeting updates (or never); now an employee sends a text message to the CEO.

Hierarchical, linear communications along the lines of an organizational chart or model no longer represent the realities of organizational activities.

A NEW ORGANIZATIONAL MODEL FOR CULTURAL EVOLUTION

In light of these advances, new organizational models are needed. These changes, resulting from innovations in digital transfer of information and communication, have rendered the organization more complex than ever before. More nimble and responsive organizational models are needed to take advantage of the digital resources and the resulting shift from work focused from primarily on operations to work in 3 spheres or a trimodal model: operations, innovation planning, and transition management. Perhaps the most important work for the innovation leader is creating this context for overall effectiveness that requires all 3 work products: operations, innovation, and transition. The innovation leader uses the trimodal organizational model to more effectively advance the work of the organization and create a context whereby creative thinking is valued, improvement is rewarded, and individuals feel safe in recommending or initiating innovative ways of working and producing outcomes. The expectation is that the workplace supports quality, creativity, new thinking, willingness to challenge long-held assumptions, and the means to transition between the current state and the desired future state. Recognition of these 3 aspects of organizational work is needed to assure survival of the organization, advancement of practices and services, integration of essential work partners, and sustainability of new ideas. The first aspect of work is traditional operations.

Operations, or the work of providing evidence-based patient care within a defined structure with supportive staff and resources, have traditionally been the focus of the majority of health care organizations, financial institutions, and policy overseers. The majority of work and work products are planned, funded, and evaluated within the operations model. In essence, this is the technical work of an organization, provided by highly skilled professionals. The contemporary leader has learned to balance and support multiple operational entities and initiatives; medical-surgical services, ambulatory services, pharmacy services, and so forth. The new work, with greater variability and complexity, requires a shift from an emphasis on operations to a model that values and integrates the 3 distinct work products, namely traditional operations, innovation management, and the transition between operations and innovation. It is unclear as to what the exact proportion of effort should be for each of these modes; however, it is clear that less time will be spent in operations, with increasing attention to innovation and transition to new levels of operational work. The emphasis by operations on high-reliability organizations is now tempered with the notion of focus and accountability on the work being done, with the understanding that procedures necessarily will change; standardization and consistency must be continually challenged as new information and technologies are introduced. This is not to negate the importance or value of stability, rather to recognize the temporary nature of it. The emphasis must not be on completing high-reliability checklists and redundancies; the emphasis, or *time out*, is about assuring that the work about to be done is appropriate. The second aspect of work in the trimodal model is innovation planning.

Innovation planning. Innovation work is quite different from operations work. Whereas quality and stability are the goals for operations work, managing innovation planning focuses on high intensity, with continual introduction and evaluation of new ideas. Stability is anathema to innovation planning. Innovation work considers any and all new technologies and processes as potential opportunities to advance and strengthen the work of the organization. The development of new approaches to health care that are safer, less invasive, and more cost-effective occurs using the tools of innovation. The tools of innovation provide structure and rigor for these processes to assure thorough consideration, testing, and pricing. Numerous tools, spaces, and processes have been used to accomplish comprehensive evaluations. Many organizations have created physical space for this work; however, the emphasis is more on thinking differently, researching available technologies and the needs of clients. This thinking work does not require a specific physical space, rather physical or virtual space that supports creative, safe, and respectful dialog.[2]

The topics for innovation planning result from both new ideas and current ineffective or poorly functioning processes. While newly developed technologies are frequently evaluated in innovation planning, it is also the crises of organizational work that provide opportunities for course corrections and new approaches. When organizations are faced with fewer resources, negative outcomes, or shortages of workers, the innovation planning team can employ the tools of innovation to address these challenges. In this way, organizations move from being in perpetual crisis mode to that of course correction using innovative processes.[4] Crisis are quickly transformed into opportunities. Unexpected events are seldom a cause for panic, rather opportunities for improvement.

Transition work for cultural transformation. Once new ideas are identified and determined to be fit for future work within the organization, sustainable pathways to modify roles, competencies, infrastructure, technology, funding, and the cultural norms must also evolve. The significance and complexity of facilitating and assuring an effective transition between innovation and operations is often overlooked or at best underestimated. The work of changing the culture requires much more than a single educational program. When innovations are introduced into a traditional culture without adequate transition support and modification of the existing work, the innovations are most likely to be considered fads and dismissed quickly. New ideas are considered burdens rather than opportunities to remain competitive and achieve the highest quality outcomes. In many ways, the recent Carnegie Foundation National Study of Nursing Education recommendations can be integrated into this transition work to advance the cultural shift.[5] The work of transition facilitators begins with the recognition of 3 components of professional education that include cognitive knowledge, practice know-how, and ethical comportment and formation. Transition work necessarily becomes more defined, formalized, and focused when all 3 components are considered. Participants are more likely to engage in new work at higher levels when they know the rationale for change, are able to test the knowledge in practice, and can support the ethical expectations for professional practice, namely involvement in change and advancement of one's discipline. Participation in innovation work is not optional; it is the obligation of the professional to advance practice and provide feedback specific to the effectiveness and value of the new work. Again, transition is about cultural transformation and requires time, reinforcement, and frequent course corrections to successfully embed new practices into the evolving culture.

The following competencies are the hallmarks for innovation leaders, and include individual and team competencies.

INDIVIDUAL INNOVATION LEADERSHIP COMPETENCIES

Assessment for innovation. Internal or personal knowledge about one's propensity, skills, and abilities with innovation work begins the developmental journey for traditional leaders. The more clearly an individual understands personal perspectives, motives, and styles, the greater potential for effective communication and the advancement of innovation. The focus for the innovation leader is to begin transformation with oneself; revolutionizing health care from the inside out, beginning with a clear understanding of personal beliefs and behaviors. The ability to understand and learn from others and collaborate with multiple styles in multidisciplinary teams is the ultimate goal of the innovation leader.

Awareness of style and innovation tendencies relate specifically to the following.

- *Personal reflection and ego management.* Individuals often get stuck in work processes that insulate and sometimes blind them to the opportunities and changes emerging in their environment. The innovation leader periodically sets time aside to reflect on work routines, challenge assumptions, and think about how work might be done differently or might even be eliminated. Challenging assumptions and thinking differently need not be a complicated or formal process, rather simply selecting an activity or routine, and taking 15 to 20 minutes to examine it and create new possibilities to share with one's team. For the overscheduled leader, reserving time for future thinking may be the most critical and courageous step taken. As innovation competence develops, the innovation leader is less and less tempted to direct and manage things and people, and the emphasis shifts to behaviors that facilitate and empower the performance of others. This awareness also includes willingness to correct a course quickly when one idea or project does not yield the desired results.
- *Appreciative inquiry style.* The work is about facilitating and empowering others rather than directing and doing; it is about understanding others using multiple strategies and approaches. The leader transcends the tacit knowledge management of knowing what and why to do something to self-transcend knowledge. The leader moves from reliance on historical knowledge to imagining, intuiting, inspiring, and reflecting the present as the means to the future.[3]
- *Courage to confront* and an awareness of personal vulnerability to see differing perspectives and values not as conflict, but rather as opportunities for new ideas and insights. This attitude includes the courage to challenge assumptions and ask difficult questions as the means to explore new ideas and assure continuous value of work processes, eliminating obsolete health care dogma, and not being derailed by the criticism or ridicule that might occur. The goal is to thrive in challenging the status quo, to not be fearful or reluctant to continually validate even the most basic work. Courage is essential in outwardly recognizing the need to move forward and beyond the status quo.
- *Emotional competence propensities.* The relationship between emotions and intellectual content is important in understanding not only one's personal style but also the abilities of others. Emotional competence that is steeped in passionate optimism for the future and impulse control serves the innovation leader well.
- *Decision-making considerations* using creativity and open dialog. Knowledge of decision-making, communication, and conflict resolution styles are helpful assessments for this role. Myers Briggs (see http://www.myersbriggs.org/) and DISC (see http://www.profiles4u.com/what-is-disc-profile.asp) assessments are examples of these assessment tools for individuals.
- *Processing of information* emphasizing "big picture" thinking, tolerance for ambiguity, and uncertainty of details. Awareness of information-processing styles and thinking systems styles as a means to excel as transformational leaders is necessary. Consideration is also given to understanding rational and experiential

information-processing styles.[7] Rational processing is analytical, intentional, logical, and slower, whereas experiential information processing is holistic, automatic, associative, and faster. The innovation leader necessarily requires both modes of processing to be effective.

- *Expressions of innovation* similar to the faces of innovation. Kelly's Ten Faces of Innovation[6] describe the personas and different approaches to new ideas.
- *Courage to stretch performance.* Innovation leaders see prodigious possibilities in the future and engage others to advance work, emphasizing the processes of work rather than the individual behaviors. Courage is also about creating stretch goals, rather than "hunkering down" in economic downturns, to advance the breadth and depth of the organization. This approach focuses on sustaining the past and present. Note that the decision to "hunker down" assumes there is excess capacity, whereby the possibility exists to tighten one's belt and cut costs to allow the organization to grow.

Future-focused. The innovation leader tends to be future oriented, actively planning for a better future. The innovation leader is constantly aware of the inevitability and value of change. This leader constantly scans changes in the external environment, technology, new processes, and others' innovations to determine their impact on the internal environment. This predictive and adaptive leadership work helps keep team members in the workplace constantly aware of circumstances and conditions that may influence and challenge the staff and the work they do.

Value-driven. Closely linked to the future orientation of the innovation leader is the expectation that new ideas will advance performance and value to the key stakeholders. Changes to the work of the organization necessarily must increase the value of the defined mission. The tools of innovation and the business case for innovation are helpful in assuring the innovation work is clearly defined and then examined from the business value perspective.

The tools of innovation, as previously noted, are helpful for several reasons. First, the tools guide individuals in using reliable methods for knowledge assessment and creation, and second, assist in discriminating innovation work from operations. The innovation leader recognizes that innovation planning and leadership require different ways of communicating, interacting, processing ideas, and thinking to accomplish the work of innovation planning. Knowledge of the concepts and the tools of innovation as well as being technologically inquisitive are essential for the innovation leader. Examples of the tools of innovation include scenario planning, deep-dive experiences, innovation labs, virtual innovation models, and brainstorming.[1,2] Providing new opportunities and new tools for stimulating ideas along with the conversations and deliberations that give these ideas form, substance, and direction is the new work of innovation planning.

In addition to innovation tools, creating the business case for innovation[8] becomes an essential step in advancing innovation work. The lack of historical data or experience to document expected returns on innovation investment does not negate the need for sound business rationale for any new resource expenditure. There are 10 elements to include in an innovation proposal (**Box 1**). Documentation of this information then forms the background data for traditional business planning formats when the work is moved into operations.

Innovation-focused team behaviors. Teamwork in an innovation-sensitive culture requires individuals with high self-awareness, external biases for innovation and behaviors that focus on learning from others, facilitation of progress, and minimal

---

Box 1
Business case for innovation: essential elements

1. Description of the product or service

2. Purpose of the product or service

3. Projection of costs required to launch the innovation

4. Costs excluded from the proposal and rationale for exclusion

5. Projection of benefits and evidence for the anticipated benefits

6. Timeline for development and launching of innovation

7. Anticipated profit or loss for at least 3 years

8. Other benefits anticipated to include community benefit, reputation, and satisfaction of clients

9. Anticipated risks and plans to mediate the risks

10. Summary of short-term and long-term value to all stakeholders

---

extolling of personal goals, competencies, and virtues. The following rules of engagement for innovation teams guide all members of the team.

Once individuals have developed competence with innovation behaviors, the next step is innovation teamwork: multiple individuals competent with innovation behaviors working together. Team expectations personify and extend self-knowledge, including avoidance of judgment, limiting ideas, prejudice, and historic ways of working. In the team setting, the goal is to bring together individuals who can collectively brainstorm, embrace risk-taking, and think laterally to create collective wisdom. Achieving the next brilliant plan or idea as quickly as possible occurs when there is openness and genuine encouragement of new ideas among diverse individuals. Team members, as catalysts for change, behave in ways to advance future thinking, creativity, trust, risk-taking, and mutual respect.

The following rules of engagement are recommended for both new and experienced innovation teams.

Rules of engagement for innovation teams:
1. Be courageous and vulnerable. The innovation leader continually strives to role model the state of vulnerability as comfort with uncertainty, thrives on finding solutions to difficult problems, embraces change willingly as the best vehicle for a better future, and believes innovation requires many perspectives and skills from many individuals. For the innovation leader, vulnerability is about knowing that one can never know everything there is to know. This *perpetual incompleteness* is a fundamental reality for innovation-driven individuals. All team members will role model courage to be vulnerable through activities of challenging traditional norms and practices, confronting each other when resistance is evident, taking risks. It is the courage and *openness* developed in partner communications that lays the foundation for effective courage and openness in team work. Innovation teamwork is highly focused on more than accomplishing tasks; it is about accomplishing work AND gaining new and more in-depth appreciation of the skills, experiences, and resources of all team members that advance new ideas. Risk-taking in thinking, communication, and action are normative for innovation teams.
2. Select members strategically to facilitate future thinking. Participants are selected strategically, namely key stakeholders and those with potential to

contribute to the discussions from differing perspectives. Selecting team members is more now about including widely disparate thinkers than those believed to be entitled to membership. Innovation teams often include disparate disciplines such as clinicians, engineers, computer specialists, designers, and representatives from several age generations and ethnic cultures. In fact, innovation leaders seek out those known for strong opinions, ability to challenge others, taking risks, and thinking creatively.

Of note, while the innovation leader is patient, tolerant, and interested in diverse discussion in facilitating teamwork, collaboration and consensus building is not always supported. According to Hansen,[9,10] teams can be ineffective when members collectively agree to sustain the present or past rather than select a believed more risky venture. Further collaboration for collaboration's sake may not lead to any advantages or value.

3. Engage in genuine, respectful dialog. The most challenging aspect of innovation work is the management of one's ego in group processes. Focusing on others and learning about their experiences and knowledge requires self-discipline and comfort with personal worth. Creativity emerges when individuals are respected, valued, and encouraged to share ideas. It is important to not dismiss or negate any ideas until the team fully explores the ideas and collectively determines the fit for future work. The approach using appreciation of past successes and exploring the rationale for successes supports creativity more than discussing poor outcomes and what went wrong. More can be gained in reinforcing positive work choices and processes.

4. A bias for innovation drives the work. Innovation thinkers believe there is always a better way to do work given the nature of evolving technology, processes, pharmaceuticals, materials, and resources. "Thinking big" is normative and expecting to change the world commonplace with highly functioning innovation teams. The larger system beyond current issues is within sight for innovation planners. In contrast, staying the course or "hunkering down" to save costs is not the primary focus of innovation planning—and yet, the results of innovation work may result in significant savings.

5. Expect and acknowledge individual and team growth. Debriefing will occur as the final step of each meeting to share feedback and emphasize member innovation behaviors. Using appreciate inquiry in debriefing serves to reinforce successful experiences. Questions such as "Why do you think this worked so well?," or "What would make this even better?" further support openness to new ideas and the successes of taking risks.

6. Collectively recognize less than effective results; celebrate and move on—collectively!

All team members are responsible for course correction. When things are not going well, team members examine and evaluate the situation and facilitate appropriate course correction. This course correction emphasizes learning from the experience without ascribing blame to anyone.

7. Minimize "trash-talk." The innovation team member quickly recognizes this information and respectfully moves away from discussing extremely remote possibilities that could derail creative thinking. For whatever reason, some team members are compelled to consider extremely remote and nearly irrelevant potential activities. Eliminate, or at least minimize dialog that serves no useful purpose and often derails healthy discussions and avoids facing difficult issues. Recognizing those one in a million rare possibilities or negative fantasies postpones discussion of critical issues. The minority opinion in innovation work

is often called on to move beyond consensus building when it is apparent that achieving consensus will sustain the present and obstruct movement into the future.[9] Innovation team members focus on relative problems, not irrelevant alternative options.

SUMMARY

The work of continually reengineering the infrastructure, structure, and processes for nursing practice, managing the introduction of technology, requires individuals steeped in principles of innovation, technology, evidence, and effective facilitation. The development of new ideas and transitioning into the culture is organizationally significant, and requires the full engagement and support of team members.

Moving to the future requires heightened sensitivity to digital innovations and their potential impact on health care organization structures, processes, and role behaviors. Dramatic changes in technology have forever changed the environment in which health care is delivered. Every structure, process, and caregiver has been impacted in some way, rendering existing roles and structures inadequate. The innovation lens offers a perspective to reshape structures and roles while advancing organizational excellence in a shared and meaningful way.

REFERENCES

1. Porter-O'Grady T, Malloch K. Quantum leadership: a resource for health care innovation. 2nd edition. Sudbury (MA): Jones & Bartlett; 2007.
2. Malloch K, Porter-O'Grady T. Quantum leader: a practical application for the new world of work. 2nd edition. Sudbury (MA): Jones & Bartlett; 2009.
3. Scharmer CO, Kaufer K. Universities as birthplaces for the entrepreneuring human being. Available at: http://www.ottoscharmer.com/docs/articles/2000_Uni21us.pdf. Accessed January 5, 2009.
4. Heifetz R, Grashow A, Linsky M. Leadership in a (permanent) crisis. Harv Bus Rev 2009;87:62–9.
5. Benner P, Sutphen M, Leonard-Kahn V, et al. Formation and everyday ethical comportment. Am J Crit Care 2008;17(5):473–6.
6. Kelly T. Ten faces of innovation. New York: Doubleday; 2005.
7. Cerni T, Curtis G, Colmar S. Information processing and leadership styles—constructive thinking and transformational leadership. J Leader Stud 2008;1(2):60–73.
8. BusinessLink. Use innovation to grow your business: the business case for innovation. Available at: http://www.businesslink.gov.uk/bdotg/action/detail?type=RESOURCES&:itemID=1073792537. Accessed January 5, 2009.
9. Hansen MT. When internal collaboration is bad for your company. Harv Bus Rev 2009;87:83–8.
10. Contu D. Why teams don't work. Harv Bus Rev 2009;87:99–105.

Chief Nursing Officer Turnover: An Analysis of the Literature

Joyce Batcheller, MSN, RN, NEA-BC, FAAN

KEYWORDS

• Chief nursing officer • Executive turnover • Nursing executive

The American Organization of Nurse Executives (AONE) (2006) reported from a study that approximately 62% of the Chief Nursing Officer (CNO) respondents indicated that they anticipated making a job change in less than 5 years and more than one-quarter of the CNOs who were interviewed planned to retire. A change of more than 70% in the current CNO leadership in the country has important implications for nursing.

That same study cited that the top 5 reasons for leaving a prior CNO position were taking another job, pursuing advancement or career development opportunities, conflicts with their Chief Executive Officer (CEO), job dissatisfaction, and family/personal reasons. Approximately 40% had left their CNO position at least 1 time in their career. Approximately 25% of the CNOs who left a position had been asked to resign, had their position terminated, or lost their jobs involuntarily. Those CNOs who had resigned involuntarily wished they had "someone who understood their plight" and identified that counseling and coaching would have been helpful supports.[1]

The CNO tenure was most likely to be affected when there was a conflict with the CEO. One common reason (style differences between the CEO and the CNO) was cited by Kippenbrook as early as 1995. A second area that contributes to attrition is differences in work expectations, competencies, and what the CEO and CNO believed were noteworthy contributions to the organization. Other factors most commonly reported by CNOs for leaving were related to a lack of power to make needed changes, financial instability of the organization, ethical conflicts, or differences and conflict with the medical team.[2,3] Witt Keiffer[4] reported on CNO turnover with similar results. CNOs highly agreed 72% of the time that CEO conflicts and financial issues contribute most to CNO turnover.

According to executive recruiters 3 trends influence CNO turnover: increasing complexity of the role, financial management issues, and chief operating officer transitions. In addition, the desired qualifications for CNOs are a minimum of a master's degree, 10 years of experience in management, and prior CNO experience.[5] Finding an adequate number of qualified candidates will become increasingly difficult.

Seton Family of Hospitals, 1345 Philomena Street, Suite 402, Austin, TX 78723, USA
E-mail address: jbatcheller@seton.org

Nurs Clin N Am 45 (2010) 11–31
doi:10.1016/j.cnur.2009.10.004   nursing.theclinics.com

IMPACT OF CNO TURNOVER

CNOs are responsible for (1) creating a compelling vision for the professional practice of nursing, (2) strategic thinking, (3) workforce development, (4) business planning, and (5) creating safe and reliable care. CNOs create and consolidate the framework for practice and influence the degree of innovation and excellence at every level of the nursing organization.[6]

The cost crisis in the American health care system and the focus on what is needed for health care reform require executive nurse leaders to become even more innovative and committed to excellence. CNO leadership affects the type and degree of commitment experienced by staff nurses in the health care organizations in which they are employed. CNOs with transformational leadership styles have a direct influence on staff nurses. This style of leadership serves to engage members of an organization, reduce feelings of alienation, and keep employee involvement productive.[7]

Five critical factors that contribute to retention of CNOs are (1) relationships with the senior leadership team, (2) authority to do the CNO job, (3) work-life balance, (4) location of the institution, and (5) the compensation package.[5] The ability to lead positive change and to make a difference was also significant to the more tenured executives.

UNIQUE ROLE/PERSPECTIVE OF THE CNO IN THE EXECUTIVE SUITE

The AONE nurse executive competencies are a description of skills that are common to nurses in executive roles. These competencies are based on a model of development established by the Healthcare Leadership Alliance in 2004. Members of this Alliance include AONE, the American College of Healthcare Executives, the Healthcare Financial Management Association, the Healthcare Information and Management Systems Society, and the Medical Group Management Association.[1] The competencies can be used as a self-assessment tool and provide guidance for job descriptions, expectations, and evaluations of nurse leaders. In addition, nurse educators can use them in curriculum development and to assist young nurse leaders with personal growth and development.[1]

CNOs are responsible for various tasks, including operations, strategies, care delivery, mentoring, and workforce management. The number 1 priority that CNOs agree is "highly important" to their success is enhancing patient care quality. Building relationships with the medical staff and aligning nursing goals with the organizational strategic plan tie as the number 2 "highly important" responsibility for their success (Appendix 1).[4]

LIMITATIONS

Finding research studies on CNO turnover and retention was a challenge. Few articles appear in the literature, yet this position is critical to the stability and movement of the organization toward better patient care.

The AONE competencies for nurse executives are a comprehensive resource. The 4 core areas of competencies are (1) communication and relationship management, (2) professionalism, (3) business skills and principles, and (4) knowledge of the health care environment.[1] Specific behaviors and skills are associated with each of these areas. One challenge may be to know which skills are needed in a prioritized manner, because it is unusual for someone to be competent in all areas when he or she begins this role.

FURTHER EXPLORATION

The challenge of finding research about the CNO role and why CNOs choose to stay or leave an organization is one nurse leaders must address. Several questions emerged from the omissions in the literature. Some of the other questions needing further exploration include:

1. What are the most critical competencies a CNO needs? Building trust and developing a strong relationship with the CEO is 1 of the most critical competencies for new CNOs to develop. Conflicts in the CEO-CNO relationship was the most commonly cited reason for CNO turnover. Relationship building is critical because the CNO must be able to create and communicate a shared vision for all levels of personnel that links the clinical and organizational goals and desired outcomes.
2. What are the unique contributions that a CNO brings to the executive suite? How can a CNO leverage these unique contributions? A CNO is in a unique position to translate how the value of nursing is essential to the success of the organization. In addition, the CNO must be able to convey this to various audiences within an organization and with relevant political stakeholders.
3. How many health care organizations use the AONE competency model for their new and current CNOs? The CNO competencies described in the AONE model are comprehensive. The self-assessment tool is likely to show different results depending on the individual's experience level. By using the self-assessment tool a CNO could gain insights into strengths he or she has that could be leveraged to enhance success. In addition, using the tool would allow an individual the opportunity to become more focused on prioritizing which skills and competencies need development to achieve the goals of the organization.
4. How many CEOs are familiar with the AONE model? Can this model serve as a tool for executives to understand their role better in supporting, mentoring, and investing in the development of a CNO? For example, if a CEO is knowledgeable about the areas that the CNO needs to develop, more focused planning can be done. Projects, experiences, mentors, and workshops could be planned together to further skill development and facilitate a person's success.
5. Are the competencies needed for a system CNO different from for a site-specific CNO? Is the ability to influence a skill more important to a system CNO because there are a greater number of stakeholders to work with? Business skills and financial management may be competencies that are even more critical to a system CNO. For example, the ability to quantify and demonstrate a return on investment may be easier with a larger number of sites than a stand-alone facility.

SUMMARY

CNOs are in a distinct position to effect transformational health care changes. Development of the current and next generation of nursing leaders to meet the needs is critical. The challenge nurse leaders face is to develop a competency model and roadmap that will assist nurse executives in becoming transformational leaders. The CNO is in a unique role to affect positively the health status and outcomes for patients. Decreasing CNO turnover through more focused CNO development and succession planning are critical areas that an organization needs to focus on.

REFERENCES

1. American Organization of Nurse Executives. AONE nurse executive competencies. Nurs Leader 2006;30(1):50–6.
2. Kippenbrook T, May F. Turnover at the top: CNOs and hospital characteristics. Nurs Manag 1994;25(9):54–7.

3. Havens DS, Thompson PA, Jones CB. Chief nursing officer retention and turnover: a crisis brewing? Results of a national study. J Healthc Manag 2008;53(2):89–106.
4. Kieffer Witt. Chief nursing officers: their role and keys to effectiveness. A confidential Witt/Kieffer survey of chief nursing officers. 2003. Available at: http://www.wittkieffer.com. Accessed July 24, 2009.
5. Havens DS, Thompson PA, Jones CB. Chief nursing officer turnover: chief nursing officers and healthcare recruiters tell their stories. J Nurs Adm 2008;38(12): 516–25.
6. Marquis BL, Houston CJ. Leadership roles and management functions in nursing: theory and application. 5th edition. Philadelphia: Lippincott Williams & Wilkins; 2005.
7. Leach L. Nurse executive transformational leadership and organizational commitment. J Nurs Adm 2005;35(5):228–37.

Appendix 1: Literature Matrix

Source	Purpose	Study Design Variables: Dependent/Independent Outcome/Endpoint	Subjects: Number of Subjects Inclusion/Exclusion	Data: Source of Instrument Data Collection Period Statistical Analysis	Results Limitations Comments
Adams C. The impact of problem-solving of nurse executives and executive officers on tenure. J Nurs Adm 1993;23(12):38–43.	To determine if CEOs and CNOs in the same hospital have the same problem-solving style. To determine if the tenure of the CNO is related to the problem-solving pair of the CEO/CNO pair	Study design: correlational Variables: independent Problem-solving style: dependent Relationship of the CEO-CNO pair	Subjects: 91 accredited acute care hospitals in Idaho, Montana, eastern Washington and eastern Oregon	Source: Citron: adaptation innovation inventory problem-solving tool Informational questionnaire for CNOs Analysis: Post hoc analysis to determine source of significance	Findings: 66 (73%) of CEO/CNO pairs responded with usable research data Scores: 24 (36%) CNOs were adaptors 42 (64%) CNOs were innovators 14 (21%) CEOs were adaptors 52 (79%) CEOs were innovators Four groups formed: CNO-CEO style: Adaptor-adaptor Adaptor-innovator Innovator-innovator Innovator-adaptor CNO/CEO pairs where both were adaptors had the longest tenure CNO tenure was shortest when the CNO was an innovator and the CEO was an adaptor CNO/CEO pairs where both were innovators did not see longer tenure Comments: High performance teams are essential to a hospital's efficiency, effectiveness, and success. CNO-CEO pairs who share similar problem-solving styles have many advantages. This kind of self-knowledge may be useful when a CNO is interviewing for a job. In addition there are strengths and limitations to each problem-solving style. It may be important to teach about those differences to gain appreciation for this kind of diverse thinking

(continued on next page)

Appendix 1:
(continued)

Source	Purpose	Study Design Variables: Dependent/Independent Outcome/Endpoint	Subjects: Number of Subjects Inclusion/Exclusion	Data: Source of Instrument Data Collection Period Statistical Analysis	Results Limitations Comments
Beyers M. The changing world of nurse administrative practice. J Nurs Adm 1995;25(2):5–6, 32.					Comments: AONE members wrote this column to raise issues and discuss trends of importance to nursing administrators
Bloudin AS, Brent NJ. Nurse administrators in job transition: stories from the front. J Nurs Admin 1992;22(12):13–4, 27.					Comments: Explores involuntary CNO turnover through interviews Discusses employment contracts as a tool for CNOs to use CNOs described their experiences as painful and at times offered relief from painful situations
Broome GH, Hughes RL. (1990) Leadership development: past, present, and future. Greensboro, NC: Center for Creative Leadership.					Comments: Changing contexts that will affect leadership development include: • globalization/internationalization of leadership concepts, constructs, and development methods • role of technology • integrity and character of leaders • demonstrate return on investment • new ways of thinking about the nature of leadership and leadership development

Citation	Purpose	Comments
Cathcart EB. The role of the chief nursing officer in leading the practice. Nurs Admin Q 2008;32(2):87–91.	Purpose: Using the Benner model, the author discusses why the CNO must create an environment within the organization for the practice to be fully lived out if he or she is to be successful as a leader of the discipline	Comments: Three lessons learned by using Benner's model include: (1) being able to access the internal goods of clinical nursing practice resets the agenda for everyone (2) being able to cull out and put language to the intentions and actions of the nurse changes the understanding and value of the work (3) being in touch with the ethical mandate of the practice can serve as a moral compass in a world fraught with tough choices
Chiverton P, Witzel P. What CNOs really want. Nurs Manage 2008;1:33–47.		Comments: Summarizes and gives examples of 5 core competencies all clinicians will need to have in the twenty-first century, which include: (1) delivering patient-centered care (2) working as a multidisciplinary team (3) practicing evidence-based medicine (4) focusing on quality improvement (5) using information technology

(continued on next page)

Appendix 1:
(continued)

Source	Purpose	Study Design Variables: Dependent/Independent Outcome/Endpoint	Subjects: Number of Subjects Inclusion/Exclusion	Data: Source of Instrument Data Collection Period Statistical Analysis	Results Limitations Comments
Del Bueno DJ. Nurse executive turnover. Nurs Econ 1993;1:25-8.	Purpose: To describe the employment patterns among nurse executives participating in the Johnson and Johnson Wharton Fellows Program	Study design: survey Variables: nurse executives who attended the Wharton Fellows Program	Enrolled = 341 fellows Inclusion: CNOs who attended the Wharton Fellows Program from all 50 states representing various ages, educational preparation, and years of experience Exclusion: non-USA fellows and individuals who report to a previous Wharton Fellow	Source: Survey of 341 CNOs who attended a 3-week residency at the Wharton Fellows Program Convenience sample of non-Fellow CNOs and a sample of their hospital administrators was used for comparison Data collection period: 1983–1992	Findings: 341 participants made 184 changes as nurse executives 217 (64%) were no longer in the same position as when they participated as a fellow Comparison to non-Wharton Fellows showed similar relationship to the number of CNOs who made no changes at all during the study period (36%) Non-Fellows have a higher overall percentage (30%) of CNOs no longer in an executive position Eight Fellows were promoted to a COO level Limitations: Selection criteria bias the sample
Dragoo J. Mentoring a novice chief nurse executive. J Nurs Admin 1998;28(9):12-4.					Comments: This article describes the potential benefits of a mentor relationship for new CNOs. The article also gave an overview of what a mentor relationship needs to be to be effective
Dubnicki C, Sloan S. Excellence in nursing management. J Nurs Admin 1991;21(6):40-5.	Purpose: To explore what characteristics are most typically demonstrated by outstanding nurse managers	Study design: structured individual interviews of nurse managers Variables:	Inclusion: Four managers were chosen from each facility The directors of each manager also participate in a questionnaire	Source: Six nationally prominent teaching hospitals in competitive geographic markets Participants:	Findings: Nine competencies that are related to 5 general groups of skills were identified as follows:

Feldman H. Preparing the nurse executive of the future. Nurs Leader Forum 1995;1(1):18–22.	nurse managers in similar nurse manager positions as described by content of job description and structure of the organization to include: • 24-hour responsibility • most time in management activities • hours are not included in patient care hours • responsible for unit budgeting	24 managers were included who were described by their directors as solid or outstanding performers	(1) achievement/getting the job done • initiative • achievement orientation (2) management/working through others • directing others • group management (3) interpersonal relationships/working with others • use of influence strategies • interpersonal sensitivity • direct persuasion (4) problem-solving • analytical thinking (5) personal performance/managing oneself • self-confidence Limitations: sample size Comments: A competency model can greatly enhance the effectiveness of the hospitals' selection and development efforts Comments: The author gives an overview of the kinds of skills a CNO will need to be successful The author advocates the need for intense collaboration between academia and practice

(continued on next page)

Appendix 1:
(continued)

Source	Purpose	Study Design Variables: Dependent/Independent Outcome/Endpoint	Subjects: Number of Subjects Inclusion/Exclusion	Data: Source of Instrument Data Collection Period Statistical Analysis	Results Limitations Comments
Fralic FM. Into the future: nurse executives and the world of information technology. J Nurs Admin 1992;22(4):11–2.					Comments: The author reviews the impact that technology can have in the clinical environment and the need for CNOs to conceptualize, justify, and plan, then integrate new systems to improve care and expert nursing management
Fralic FM. Nurse executive practice–into the next millennium: from limbo dancer to pole vaulter. J Nurs Admin 1992;22(2):15–6.					Comments: The author reviews strategies and practices (past, present and future) for their relevance, practicality, and success The author stresses the need for periodic self-assessments
Freund CM. CEO succession and its relationship to CNO tenure. J Nurs Admin 1987;17(7–8):27–30.	To describe the relationship between CEO succession and CNO termination	Study design: survey Variables: independent: • CEO succession dependent: • CNO terminations	Inclusion: CEOs from 250 university-owned or -affiliated hospitals	Source: Questionnaire used in an earlier study to study tenure history of CNOs Time period: 1973–1982	Findings: CEO reasons for leaving: • termination 24 (25.3%) • retirement 16 (16.8%) • promotion 12 (12.6%) • other 12 (12.6%) • personal 8 (8.4%) • job dissatisfaction 8 (8.4%) • no reason given 15 (15.8%) CEOs on average enjoy longer tenure and are not so susceptible to separation by request or mandates as CNOs Comments: At least 12% of CNO terminations can be accounted for by the

Reference	Aim/Purpose	Study design	Inclusion/Data/Limitations	Findings/Comments
Hader R. Are you prepared for your role as a CNO? Nurs Manage 2007;38(3):43–4.				Comments: The article outlines several factors that a prospective CNO should consider before assuming a role as an administrator
Hader R. Board governance: what's your CNO role? Nurs Manage 2006;37(3):32–4.				Comments: The article presents an overview of the role of the board of trustees. In addition, the article describes the role of the CNO and skills needed for a CNO to be effective
Havens DS, Thompson PA, Jones CB. Chief nursing officer turnover: chief nursing officers and healthcare recruiters tell their stories. J Nurs Admin 2008;38(12), 516–25.	To examine CNO turnover to inform the development of strategies to improve CNO recruitment and retention and ease transition for those who turnover	Study design: qualitative descriptive design	Inclusion: All of the CNOs who participated in the phase I survey were invited at the end of the survey to contact a study investigator if they were willing to participate in phase 2 interviews. In addition, all US hospital and health system CNOs (AONE members and nonmembers) were invited. In addition, health care executive recruiters employed in search firms known to recruit for vacant CNO positions were interviewed. Data: Individual participant interviews were contacted by 1 of the study investigators and participated in a 35- to 40-minute interview by phone. Interviewees participated from a location of their choice (work, home, or other remote site). Sample size: 26 with current and past CNOs and health care recruiters. Limitations: sample size	Findings: Informants who involuntarily resigned had 4 central themes: • hospital financial concerns • conflict between CEO and CNO • appointment of a new CEO • other concerns about CNO financial management Voluntary turnover signs of predicting what was coming: • deterioration of CEO-CNO relationship • ethical conflicts/differences • hospital fiscal health • blindsided Insights from CNOs with no turnover: • ability to lead positive change and make a difference • passion for the CNO role • mentoring and enhancing nursing practice • good relationships with the senior leadership team

(continued on next page)

Appendix 1: (continued)

Source	Purpose	Study Design Variables: Dependent/Independent Outcome/Endpoint	Subjects: Number of Subjects Inclusion/Exclusion	Data: Source of Instrument Data Collection Period Statistical Analysis	Results Limitations Comments
Jones CB, Havens DS, Thompson PA. Chief nursing officer retention and turnover: a crisis brewing? Results of a national survey. J Healthc Manage 2008;53(2):89–106.	To study the CNO dissatisfaction, intent to leave, and turnover	Study design: survey Variables: independent: • current/permanent CNOs, interim and past CNOs	Subjects: 634 CNOs: 622 (985) were in a permanent role; 12 (2%) were in an interim role	Source: Confidential online survey Time period: 4 weeks: 28 September– 28 October 2005	Insights from health care recruiters: • destabilizing environment • trust and security issues • culture of fear • quality of care • public perceptions • program inertia Five critical retention issues were: (1) relationships with senior leadership team (2) compensation package (3) authority to do CNO job (4) work-life balance (5) location of the institution Findings: CNO turnover (n = 622) Never experienced turnover—60.3% CNOs who had experienced job turnover—39.7% • turnover within past 2 years—13% • within past 2–5 years—12.4% • within past 5–10 years—8.7% • greater than 10 years—5.6% Type of turnover: • voluntary—76.5% • involuntary—23.4%

- asked to resign—8.1%
- terminated—4.4%
- other reasons—10.9%

Top reasons for prior turnover (n = 247)

- take another CNO position—49.8%
- promotion or career advancement—28.7%
- conflicts with CEO—25. %
- job dissatisfaction—20.6%
- family/personal reasons—20.2%

Major concern is that 61% of respondents anticipate a job change in less than 5 years

Limitations:

Survey was anonymous, so it did not allow for individual respondents to be tracked nor control of the number of times a participant responded

Comments:

The need for succession planning for CNOs is evident from this study

AONE believes these 4 specific policy issues need to be addressed:

(1) services needed for nurse executives who experience involuntary turnover

(2) support for leadership succession planning

(3) continuing and supplemental education programs

(4) characteristics of work/practice environment for nursing leadership

(continued on next page)

Appendix 1:
(continued)

Source	Purpose	Study Design Variables: Dependent/Independent Outcome/Endpoint	Subjects: Number of Subjects Inclusion/Exclusion	Data: Source of Instrument Data Collection Period Statistical Analysis	Results Limitations Comments
Kippenbrook T, May F. Turnover at the top: CNOs and hospital characteristics. Nurs Manage 1994; 25(9):54–7.	Purpose To describe institutional factors influencing CNO turnover To compare CNO turnover to CEO turnover To determine if CNO turnover has changed in the past 5 years	Study design: retrospective descriptive data Variables: • CNO turnover • hospitals with CNO and CEO turnover in the same year • type of hospital ownership	Subjects: 102 randomly selected urban and rural hospitals	Data: Turnover data collected from: Hospital Blue Book Directory of Hospital Personnel Institutional data collected from: Guide to the Health Care Field Data collection period: 5-year period (1987–1992) Relationship between hospital characteristics and CNO turnover using t-tests, χ^2 testing, Pearson product moment correlation and analysis of variance found 2 significant findings	Results: The 102 hospitals in this sample experienced 110 CNO turnovers during the study period No CNO turnover in 29 hospitals, 1 turnover in 44 of the hospitals Annual CNO turnover ranged from 14.7% to 27.5% between 1998 and 1992 Highest CNO turnover in 1990 and 1991 Average CNO turnover = 21.6% Only 9% of hospitals had the same CNO and CEO during the entire 5-year period of the study Findings: CNOs departed more frequently from hospitals with lower occupancy rates and more frequently from rural hospitals than from urban hospitals Comments: Hospitals with lower occupancy rates and in rural communities continue to have the most financial challenges in today's competitive environment Characteristics of successful CNOs, including those with longevity, need to be studied in an effort to enhance retention

	Study design: descriptive design using a survey approach	Inclusion:	Findings:
Kippenbrook, T. Turnover of hospital chief nursing officers. Nurs Econ 1995;13(6):330–6. To examine factors contributing to chief nursing officer turnover	Variables: independent: • CNOs who left their job in the past year • CEOs for whom the CNOs had worked dependent: • departure • performance • relationships • demographics	• potential subjects were identified by full-time CNO changes between 1992 and 1993 • hospital CEO for whom the CNO had worked during the same time frame	Results: • 68 CNO questionnaires returned for a 40% participation rate • 47 CEOs for a 28% response rate CNO demographics: • 93% female, mean age was 48 and 62% were married with children • highest nursing degree earned was 17% ADN, 30% BSN, 26% Masters, 2% Doctoral and 25% Diploma CEO demographics: • 72% male with a mean age of 49 • highest degree: masters 45% Average tenure: • CNO tenure was 5.5 years with a range from 1 to 22 years and 1–3 years the most frequent tenure. • average CEO tenure was 7 years Reasons for turnover: CNOs reported: voluntary resignation–45%, retirement–22%, termination–15%, promotion–13%lateral transfer in same organization–10% and better job offer–10%

(continued on next page)

Appendix 1:
(continued)

Source	Purpose	Study Design Variables: Dependent/Independent Outcome/Endpoint	Subjects: Number of Subjects Inclusion/Exclusion	Data: Source of Instrument Data Collection Period Statistical Analysis	Results Limitations Comments
					Professional reasons for leaving: • CNOs reported: lack of power to make changes–54%, conflicts with CEO–47%, inadequate nursing personnel–42%, changing health care system–36%, and difficulty developing an effective management team–32%, financial instability of organization–30%, desire for a better position–23%, and conflict with the medical team–21% • CEOs reported their CNOs left because of insufficient leadership/management skills–36%, changing health care environment–36%, difficulty developing an effective management team–3%, lack of perceived power–30%, conflict with CEO–30%, inadequate nursing personnel–30%, conflict with medical staff–26%, too much conflict with other hospitals–19% Comments: • compatibility of work requirement with person's role is critical for retention and job satisfaction

Citation	Purpose	Study design	Inclusion/Screened	Source	Findings
Leslie J (2003) Leadership skills and emotional intelligence. Greensboro, NC: Center for Creative Leadership.	Purpose To study the relationship between a lack of emotional intelligence and career derailment	Study design: survey	Inclusion: 302 managers attending a Center for Creative Leadership meeting	Source: BarOn emotional quotient inventory Participants were on average 42.7 years old 73% were male 81% were white 90% had a minimum of a bachelor's degree Time period: July and September 2000	Findings: Ratings on problems with interpersonal relationships were associated with low impulse control individuals who are unaware of their own emotions and are viewed as more likely to derail because of problems dealing with people • wide gap between CNO and CEO's performance evaluations suggests different work expectations, competencies, and noteworthy contributions to organization
O'Neil E, Morjikian R, Cherner D. Developing nursing leaders: an overview of trends and programs. J Nurs Admin 2008;38(4):178–83.	To gain a better understanding of the current demand and supply of nursing leadership development programs	Study design: telephone survey	Screened: CNOs, associate directors for 20 sites, deans or department chairs (16), and nurse leaders in state and local public health (18)	Source of instrument: survey using a 3-point scale from not important to absolutely mission critical. Questions based on the Center for Health Professions at University of California, San Francisco, health care leadership domains of purpose, personal, people and process and 5–6 specific competencies under each domain. Time period: Late 2005 and early 2006	Findings: List of highest competencies identified by nurse and nonnurse leaders are the following, with values in parentheses for scale of 1–3: Nurse leaders' top 5 competencies: • building effective teams (2.9) • translating vision into strategy (2.85) • communicating vision and strategy internally (2.8) • managing conflict (2.8) • managing focus on patient and customer (2.8) Nonnurse leaders' top 5 competencies: • building effective teams (2.95) • communicating vision and strategy internally (2.95)

(continued on next page)

Appendix 1:
(continued)

Source	Purpose	Study Design Variables: Dependent/Independent Outcome/Endpoint	Subjects: Number of Subjects Inclusion/Exclusion	Data: Source of Instrument Data Collection Period Statistical Analysis	Results Limitations Comments
					• translating vision into strategy (2.9) • bringing creativity to vision and strategy formation (2.85) • managing focus on patient and customer (2.8) Comments: Nursing represents the largest human resource expenditure in most case settings but it is undercapitalized in most institutions
Sanders LS, Bowcutt M. CEO/CNO relationships: survey findings. Healthc Exec 2004;19(5):22–6.	To review how CEOs and CNOs experience the relationship they have with each other	Study design: survey	Inclusion: 1000 CEOs and 776 CNOs who were members of ACHE and AONE, respectively	Source: Comparable questionnaires were faxed	Findings: 99% CEOs and 95% CNOs report that their relationship with each other is good Three out of 4 CNOs report to the CEO; most of the remainder report to the Chief Operating Officer Only 40% of CNOs report at every board meeting Most concerning finding was the perceived lack of career advancement. Although result may seem negative, it was noted that a CNO position is considered the pinnacle of a nursing career Limitations: Is a select group, because survey included only CEOs and CNOs belonging to both organizations Comments: Opportunity for CNOs to report to the board is an area that needs

Smith PM, Parsons RJ, Murray BP, et al. The new nurse executive: an emerging role. J Nurs Admin 1994;24(11): 56–62.

to be explored

Emphasize career options CNOs may have. For example, system level roles versus 1 site

Would be useful to broaden survey's scope and sample

Comments:

The author reviewed 80 articles about CNOs that were published between 1987 and 1993

The attributes identified as most essential for CNOs were outlined in a matrix

Overall this review suggests that CNOs must have a blend of clinical, business, and personal skills

Consensus was achieved that the following are essential

- the CNO must be a hospital representative in community public relations
- the CNO must have a degree in nursing and administration or business and at least 4–5 years of nursing management experience
- the CNO's pay should be equal to CEO and other positions that are comparable
- CEO and CNO must have frequent contact and have a relationship that is in the spirit of 2 coworkers striving toward the same goal, rather than a manager-employee basis

(continued on next page)

Appendix 1:
(continued)

Source	Purpose	Study Design Variables: Dependent/Independent Outcome/Endpoint	Subjects: Number of Subjects Inclusion/Exclusion	Data: Source of Instrument Data Collection Period Statistical Analysis	Results Limitations Comments
Vautier AF (1996) Critical attributes of success and derailment in the chief nursing officer role. Unpublished doctoral dissertation, Columbia University, New York.	Purpose: To study critical attributes associated with success and derailment in the CNO role	Study design: descriptive study Variables: independent: perception of environmental, job, and personal attributes	Enrolled = CNOs and CEOs employed in all size acute care hospitals throughout the United States Inclusion: a total of 214 questionnaires were mailed to CNOs and CEOs	Source: Investigator-designed critical attribute survey with a mixed sampling design Time period: Within 12 weeks from initial mailing Limitations: Replication is needed to refine the survey instrument further and use a larger sample size. Simultaneously answering success and derailment questions may have been confusing or caused bias in answers Suggest splitting into 2 separate surveys	Findings: Overall response rate was 36% (156 questionnaires) but 14 were incomplete, so final sample was 142 CEO response rate was 23% Thirteen critical attributes were suggested as more important for CNO success which include: • 3 environmental: environment that is stable, not unionized, without CEO turnover, stable financial performance, and effective cost containment • 3 job attributes: participation and strategic visioning of entire hospital, guidance of human resource management, and commitment to the success of hospital, not just to nursing. • 6 personal attributes: Ethical, integrity, honest, and dependable characteristics most important Creates a vision and is willing to take risks to fulfill the vision Strong interpersonal relationship skills, including sense of humor, sensitivity, and team player Characteristics contributing to

Citation	Purpose	Study design	Subjects	Data	Environmental / Job attributes / Findings
Witt/Keiffer (2006) How VHA chief nursing officers view their role and keys to their effectiveness. Available at: http://www. wittkieffer.com. Accessed July 24, 2009.	Purpose: To understand current compensation and benefits. In addition, to determine the most pressing challenges facing Veterans Health Administration CNOs and effectiveness in both the overall health care environment and within their organization	Study design: electronic survey	Subjects: 1136 CNOs nationwide Response rate was 308 (27%)	Data: 321 CNOs participated and 165 submitted complete data	Environmental: CEO turnover is a significant factor that influences CNO turnover Job attributes: CNO management of only the nursing department rather than the whole, more results oriented than politically oriented, no strong internal peer relations 4 personal attributes: Style of interacting is someone that is not a "people person" but an autocrat Findings: • CNOs view setting a vision but do not see themselves as successful in doing so • role in finance and organizational profitability rank lowest on CNO self-performance list • disagreements with CEO and financial issues (65%) were identified as contributing factors in CNO turnover • CNOs believe they are less successful at fostering physician-nurse relationships • 77% believe they have a lack of visibility in organization • 52% believe they have gained respect and only 33% have been successful in enhancing clinical outcomes • Work-life balance is major factor when deciding to leave profession • 2 of 3 Veterans Health Administration CNOs have no identified mentor or succession plan in place to succeed them

Contemporary Nurse Executive Practice: One Framework, One Dozen Cautions

Maryann F. Fralic, RN, DrPH, FAAN[a,b,*]

KEYWORDS

• Leadership • Management • Nurse executives
• Operational behavior • Executive behavior

Where and how does one begin to examine today's incredibly complex health care environment? Hamel and Breen[1] describe the environment of day-by-day, moment-by-moment changes, the constantly shifting realties, the unprecedented harsh challenges as one of "head snapping change."

NEW CONTEXT, NEW IMPERATIVES?

How does today's nurse executive function effectively within this new context? Does it require different skills, new competencies, and new behaviors? Can nurse executives who have always been successful in the past, irrespective of setting, move forward with the same strategic and operational behaviors? Is there "new work" associated with a new context for executive practice? To answer these questions, consider a sampling of contemporary issues: measurable and publicly reported cost-quality performance; stringent and often nonnegotiable expectations of clinical excellence; highly protocolized care; outcomes-based reimbursement systems; incredibly complex and challenging technologies; evidence-based management and evidence-based clinical care; comparative effectiveness research (both clinical and financial); unprecedented focus on productivity; aggressive capacity management and patient throughput mandates; the expectation of experimental, affordable, and sustainable care delivery models; complex and challenging manpower planning;

Selected concepts are expanded from "The CNO's World, 2009," The Nursing Executive Center of The Advisory Board Company, Washington, DC.
[a] Department of Health Systems and Outcomes, Johns Hopkins University School of Nursing, 525 North Wolfe Street, Room 528, Baltimore, MD 21205-2110, USA
[b] The Nursing Executive Center of the Advisory Board Company, 2445 M Street, NW Washington, DC 20037, USA
* Department of Health Systems and Outcomes, Johns Hopkins University School of Nursing, 525 North Wolfe Street, Room 528, Baltimore, MD 21205-2110.
E-mail address: mfralic@son.jhmi.edu

sagging institutional investment portfolios; bundled payments and stringent nonnegotiable financial expectations. One can add to this the looming untold and unknowable challenge of a health care system undergoing dramatic change.

NEW WORK?

Today's nurse leaders everywhere will face severe challenges that are distinctly unique. This will occur whether those leaders find themselves in new or existing positions. The work is rapidly changing. The response is to retool executive practice in distinct ways.

It may be helpful, in addition to acquiring new competencies and skills, to consider the advice presented by Goldsmith[2] in his insightful book. Goldsmith's[2] focus is behavioral, isolating those behaviors that increase executive effectiveness, and identifying transactional flaws that are things one should stop doing. This is in contrast to the plethora of books that promote what executives should be doing, an important distinction.

NEW CONTEXT, NEW CONCEPTUAL FRAMEWORK

It may be useful to conceptualize the challenging work of today's nurse executive as follows:

- Representing the organization's largest clinical discipline with integrity, intellect, professionalism, and an abiding commitment to excellence in patient care.
- Frequently leading major clinical and nonclinical areas throughout the organization.
- Addressing deadly serious concrete issues that often present in abstract or obtuse forms.
- Simultaneously identifying the myriad complex patterns at play.
- Frequently moving from strategy to operations, back to strategy, all within a fast-paced, seemingly nonstop milieu.
- All occurring within the context of an often unstable, always evolving, and at times overtly chaotic environment.

Many nurse executive colleagues have validated the accuracy of this depiction of their contemporary world, replete with major challenges. In addition to up-skilling their competencies and assessing their executive behaviors, the following cautions are warranted for nurse executives in every sector and every setting.

ONE DOZEN CAUTIONS
The Escalating Drumbeat for Nonstop Creativity, Innovation, and Efficiency in Patient Care

Nurse executives recognize these examples: just as one strategy is operationalized, it must be reworked; the care delivery model that was recently designed must adjust to even more stringent patient throughput requirements; capacity management is now paramount. In another example, the nursing manpower planning matrix requires that a pipeline be created to properly recruit and prepare new nurses for quality care delivery to meet the needs of the organization. Yet, present lower volumes and reduced revenues mandate that creative ways be identified to address both the near-term and long-term clinical needs of the organization, simultaneously and at lower cost. Every nurse leader can supply their own situations that depict the unavoidable "escalating drumbeat."

Wise Advice: "Stay Close to the Cash Register"

Charles Perry, a member of the National Advisory Council of the Robert Wood Johnson Executive Nurse Fellows Program, was asked for his most important piece of advice for the fellows. Without hesitation, he quoted a savvy colleague. The answer, "stay close to the cash register," was both humorous and profound.

The lesson is clear. It is absolutely essential that one know how the organization gets its money, how it spends its money, what are its financial challenges, and where lay its fiscal strengths and weaknesses. That knowledge informs proposals, presentations, and decisions. The caution is clear. Unless leaders understand their organization's "cash register" issues, they cannot be effective, influential, or successful.

Precise Quantification, Not Supplication, is the Main Allocation Determinant

Finance is the language of power in every organization. It is the language that nurse executives must learn; combined with clinical language, one becomes powerfully "bilingual," able to speak and negotiate in terms that the organization understands and respects. Supplicant language can be left behind, replaced with crisp quantification. The business case can be made, a business plan can be developed, and the likelihood of securing the requisite resources increases exponentially. The nurse executive then has an impressive voice at the table, not merely a seat. The skill of quantification has become a valued core competency of contemporary nurse executive practice.

Focus on Contribution to the Top Line, While Aggressively Managing the Bottom Line

Effective senior nurse leaders manage the bottom line with care and diligence. They meet targets, conserve resources, and rigorously analyze trends. They encourage nurse managers to consider themselves to be CEOs of a multimillion dollar clinical business unit, and to behave accordingly. They cultivate financial knowledge for themselves and for their leadership team, searching for ways to grow the bottom line.

Contemporary nurse executives also keep a close eye on opportunities to grow the top line and to make the business case. For example, serious nursing teams can redesign care delivery processes and unit staffing patterns, thereby safely increasing throughput, so that more patients can be processed in the same bed base. That is a tangible contribution to the top line, representing valuable ongoing incremental revenue.

Lead with Competency, Not with Demands

Beware of the nurse executive who figuratively "always carries the nursing flag." That person only sees the nursing perspective, only is concerned with securing nursing resources, is not viewed as a committed executive of the entire organization, and is frequently excluded from important executive suite decisions. When this happens, patients lose and nursing loses. The effective nurse leader wisely frames issues in terms of the institution's patient care mission, while acknowledging the realities and capabilities of the organization. This neutralizes and focuses any executive team discussion.

Also destructive is the nurse executive who makes demands at the executive table, such as "the X department should report to nursing." This is a great example of what Goldsmith[2] identifies as "things we should stop doing," behaviors that are interpersonally destructive. Rather, demonstrate responsibility and capability, cultivating a reputation for competence. The organization will then seek out that valuable nurse executive. When that happens, patients, the organization, and nursing all succeed.

Ultrasophisticated and Comprehensive Strategic Planning is the Watchword

A high level strategic plan is thoughtful, comprehensive, and deliberate. It is big; it is carefully developed. It takes the long view, the broad view. It provides a guide to action; a careful road map; and a vehicle for isolating, tracking, and measuring results.

A strategic plan is warranted for the challenge of nurse manpower planning in a world where there is great financial instability and an aging workforce with generational issues and erratic periods of shortage followed by periods of oversupply. An overall plan to ensure consistent excellence in clinical care is essential.

Solid predictive skills are needed, knowing that yesterday's shortage is today's surplus in some areas, yet will revert to shortage again as large numbers of valuable older experienced nurses exit the workforce in the foreseeable future. There is no certainty of exact data; the numbers for future scenarios are not available. Environmental scans and informed projections and predictions must nevertheless be made. Planning within an aura of uncertainty and mega complexity is never easy, but it is principled leadership. A comprehensive strategic manpower plan serves to guide the organization through highly unstable scenarios. Successful leaders always have a "plan B," and with very high volatility, a "plan C" may be indicated. The alternative is to have no plan, and that is simply not acceptable.

Many confuse the tactic of deciding how many new graduates to hire in the next graduation cycle, calling that a strategic plan for nursing manpower planning. It is not, and wise nurse executives know the difference.

Be Prepared to Accommodate to a Work World Where the Language and the Tools of Social Networking are Integral to Executive Practice

Think Tweet, Twitter, Bing, Facebook Lexicon, Podcasting, Survey Monkey, Skype, Kindle, Go2Meeting, EMags, Wikipedia, and so forth. Technology and various software products proliferate rapidly. They are an inescapable factor in today's work environment. Think how quickly and easily Twitter has been assimilated into the business environment, the clinical environment, the academic environment, and into everyday language.

Social networking is gaining in popularity at an unprecedented rate. New applications of these tools and technologies are appearing in all organizations. One can elect to ignore some, but will be required to adopt others. The new communication modalities being used in the nurse executives' work environment, and elsewhere, are clearly reshaping the contemporary workplace.

President Truman was Correct: "Not All Readers are Leaders, but All Leaders are Readers"

Truman was a simple man, not an academic, and not sophisticated; but, he was a wise man. He knew the value of having the right information and how that information fosters effective leadership. He expected people around him always to be well-informed.

Effective CEOs in organizations expect that the executive team will target appropriate readings from hard copy and on-line sources, will determine what has relevance for their organization, and will report and recommend action as appropriate. Scanning the relevant literature on an ongoing basis is an essential executive skill, especially necessary when operating within fast paced, constantly shifting environments. As the leadership team models the focus on thoughtful and targeted reading, it quietly becomes an institutional value, focused journal club discussions may begin, and targeted readings often serve as the fulcrum for leadership and staff retreats.

Soon the workplace becomes a "learning organization," and its actions and decisions are based on evidence and expert opinion. The institution's leadership is always asking, what are the trends, the best practices, the latest developments? What are the threats? What lessons are most valuable? Systematically scanning current business and professional literature detects the trends and issues necessary for appropriate and timely executive action.

Respect the Imperative and the Power of Major Nontraditional Partnerships and Interdependencies

Establishing partnerships has always been effective leadership. Leaders specifically cultivate traditional and nontraditional relationships, both formal and informal. They know the urgency of linkages with cross-disciplinary teams, essential in an era of highly collaborative clinical practice. They know that nursing at some point is the member of the team, and at other times is the leader. They engage nurses who can move easily from one to the other, because attaining desired patient outcomes is the shared goal.

No one profession can successfully deliver the requisite clinical and financial outcomes that the health system increasingly demands. No one profession can ensure the overall safety and quality of patient care, and at a sustainable cost level. The most successful nurse executives build thoughtful coalitions to achieve the necessary clinical, operational, and financial outcomes that very challenging environments increasingly demand. Multidisciplinary partnerships are essential and foundational to achieving excellence in patient care delivery systems.

The Forgetting Curve may Trump the Learning Curve

When there is an overwhelming burden of new information that must be processed and assimilated (as in the current work world of the nurse executive), one must first very selectively discard old information that is no longer useful. For example, one may carry around very firm ideas about how care delivery models must be designed, because those ideas have been valued for a very long time. There is the real risk, however, that they may preclude innovative thinking about the characteristics that today's models must have, in keeping with the new health care context. Some long-held ideas can impact the assimilation of new concepts. The objective is to move away from "what was" to the focus on "what can be."

A very useful mental exercise may be to acknowledge the huge bolus of new information that must be assimilated (the challenge of the learning curve), and then to mentally discard selected old information that may be impeding innovation and creativity (the forgetting curve).

There is a Relevant Science Called the Life Cycle of Organizations

Organizations have distinct life cycles; they evolve and change over the years. There are periods of growth, periods of building, periods of retrenchment, periods of decline, and periods of maintaining a stable state.

These may be precipitated by various factors, such as revenue decline, reimbursement changes, census increase or decrease, new competitors, a loss of important providers and professionals, a change in major donors, a change "at the top," and loss of an important service line. Things happen that change organizations in dramatic ways, and these changes can occur rather quickly.

As an example, a person may have been a really "good fit" for the organization as it grew and prospered. They built programs well, they thrived in that environment. They loved hiring the right people who can enhance professional practice and "grow the business." Now they find themselves in that same organization going through serious retrenchment, and they no longer are a good match. It is a time of layoffs, and cutting programs, something they do not do well. In these scenarios, "the work" of the nurse executive changes dramatically. Successful leaders periodically assess their "goodness of fit" when their organization moves into a different life cycle. A serious caution is that organizations require different types of leadership to match the demands of their changing life cycles.

The Fantasy of Work-Life Balance Versus the Discipline of Personal Energy Management

In this last caution, and perhaps the most important, two common sense approaches are offered. First, many busy professionals seem to be chasing the fantasy of having perfect balance between their personal and professional lives. New concepts are emerging, however, that are very encouraging. Hammonds[3] reassures that perfect balance is an illusion, never quite attainable for more than a brief time. Just when someone thinks they have it, something happens to change it all, and that is the nature of reality.

People are urged to be aware that everyone has a changing "portfolio of responsibilities," and that perpetual change is inevitable, so one must respond, making necessary adjustments. Hammonds[3] encourages the reader to answer one question, "Are you happy?" Those who say yes are in balance, liberating indeed.

A second approach, by Loehr and Schwartz,[4] wisely admonishes one to pay less attention to managing time, and more attention to managing energy. Time is finite, it cannot be renewed; all have the same 24-hour box. Energy, however, can be replenished as one discards activities, actions, and responsibilities that one has assumed, but can be done by others; or can be done at another time or in a different way; or need not be done at all. When one consciously applies this mental screen, opportunities for the creation of new energy become available.

One's individual energy level is a precious personal resource. It is indeed powerful in that it is the indispensable factor that enables one to be successful, and it must be carefully guarded. It is essential to realize that in highly unstable and demanding environments, as nurse executive responsibilities inevitably expand, keen attention to self-care becomes even more crucial.

Personal energy management is a discipline that all highly successful executives cultivate; it is their lifeline. Loehr and Schwartz[4] state that it is "the key to high performance and personal renewal." As personal energy is consciously and systematically replenished, leaders are able to fully engage in their work world, and to look forward to using their skills to address the unprecedented clinical and financial challenges and complexities that lie ahead. All the while, the pursuit of excellence is the nonnegotiable goal, bringing a new level of engagement and satisfaction to the "new work" of the contemporary nurse executive.

REFERENCES

1. Hamel G, Breen B. The future of management. Boston: Harvard Business School Press 2007;39(9):2.
2. Goldsmith M. What got you here won't get you there: how successful people become even more successful. New York: Hyperion 2007;38(7/8):322–24.
3. Hammonds KH. Balance is bunk. Fast Company 2004; 68–76. Available at: http://www.fastcompany.com/magazine/87/balance1.html. Accessed April, 2009.
4. LoehrJ, Schwartz T. The power of full engagement: managing energy, not time, is the key to high performance and personal renewal. New York: Press 2003; 37(2):72.

Coaching: An Effective Leadership Intervention

Margo A. Karsten, RN, BSN, MSN, PhD

KEYWORDS

• Leadership competencies • Executive coaching
• Humanistic approach • Management

Anyone working in leadership is seeing a dramatic shift in what type of competencies are now being required to be effective. In health care, where change is the norm, it is becoming very clear that if leaders do not learn a different way of leading, turnover rates will continue to increase, and patient satisfaction and employee and physician engagement will continue to decrease. As health-care reform is on the horizon, how can leaders create organizations that are as adaptable and resilient as they are focused and efficient? Leaders need a new way of being.

LITERATURE REVIEW

According to Anderson,[1] we are breaking from traditional paternal bureaucratic forms of organizations to high-involvement, empowered-partnership, and collaborative-learning organizations. These changes will take a new set of competencies from our leaders. As we pass from the old era of morally deficient and redundant management philosophies, we are faced with the need for a new paradigm. Rampant materialism, consumption, and rationalism are giving way to a new humanistic approach rooted in values.[2] As a nation, we are moving out of the industrial era and into an era that values balance, respect, and meaningful work. According to Hamel,[3] managers must first admit that they have reached the limits of management 1.0: the industrial-age paradigm built atop the principles of standardization, specialization, hierarchy, and control. Second, they must cultivate, rather than repress, their dissatisfaction with the status quo. Third, managers need the courage to aim high.

Leading this type of transformation requires the ability to relate and influence people to accomplish extraordinary things. Specific to health care, Koloroutis[4] states that leaders at all levels of the organization play a vital role in the design and implementation of the patient-care delivery system and in creating and sustaining the culture to support it. Caring and compassionate service evolves from caring and compassionate leaders.

Faculty Member at University of Colorado, 1268 Falcon Court, Windsor, CO 80550, USA
E-mail address: mk@thecontemplativelife.org

Nurs Clin N Am 45 (2010) 39–48
doi:10.1016/j.cnur.2009.11.001   **nursing.theclinics.com**
0029-6465/10/$ – see front matter © 2010 Elsevier Inc. All rights reserved.

Given that caring competencies have not been listed as critical skills to have in the executive suite, the challenge is learning how to shift the old way of leading into a new way of being. Block[5] noticed that most people involved in culture change were unaware of their own contribution to the problems in the culture and were busy blaming others. The organizational challenge is to introduce a new way of leading. According to Hamel, managers today face a new set of problems and he cites the following problems as the most critical:

> How in a world where the winds of creative destruction blow at gale force can a company innovate quickly and boldly enough to stay relevant and profitable? How in a creative economy where entrepreneurial genius is the secret to success do you inspire employees to bring the gifts of initiative, imagination, and passion to work every day? What's needed are daring goals that will motivate a search for radical new ways of mobilizing and organizing human capabilities.[3]

As reform is looming on the horizon, these are pertinent questions for health-care leaders to ask.

Such radical change must be embraced. One intervention that assists in leadership change is coaching. Executive coaching is an intervention that is commonly implemented in business settings. Coaching provides a space for profound personal development and enables managers to understand how to translate personal insights into improved effectiveness and ultimately organizational development (Wales, 2002).[6] Organizations utilize coaches to focus on achieving specific results related to an individual's tolerance and response to emerging trends, including complexity in organizations, rapidly changing technology, and the need for enhanced processes in making decisions (Weber, 2005).[7] Further, coaching is a way to provide leaders with necessary tools and support to excel in their current role and to gain a sense of self awareness that allows them to enhance their effectiveness and relationships with people in the workplace. Evidence is beginning to suggest that corporate-level coaching offers an effective method of supporting leaders to develop a culture of innovations.[8] In fact, coaching may be capable of creating an impact at all levels of the organization and of modifying its genetic code.[9]

Based on literature, coaching seems to be an effective strategy in transforming leaders and cultures. With limited resources, health-care executives need to ask: is the cost of coaching worth the organizational commitment and investment? In one of the first empirical studies of the effects of coaching, training alone accounted for a 22.4% increase in productivity, but when followed with coaching, productivity increased 88%.[10] Thach[11] utilized a 360-degree feedback instrument to determine the impact of executive coaching on leadership effectiveness. Two hundred and eighty one leaders participated in 360-degree feedback before and after an average of 6 months of coaching. The overall impact of leadership effectiveness, as perceived by direct reports, peers, and managers, was an average of 55% and 60% respectively during the two phases of the study.[11] Lastly, Laske[12] investigated the mental and emotional growth of six executives who were coached over 14 months. Coaches' and participants' developmental and behavioral profiles were assessed before and after coaching. Three executives made significant developmental progress and were perceived to have improved their leadership effectiveness through the use of coaching.[12]

It is evident that a leadership shift is needed within health care. Based on multiple studies, coaching appears to be a systematic leadership intervention that will lead to a radical cultural change. Coaching is evolving as a practical, cost-effective, and evidence-based organizational method for assisting leaders to improve their performance in areas of leadership, communication, and productivity.

CASE STUDY

In 2003, like most health-care organizations, a hospital in the western region of the country was experiencing great transition. Multiple chief executive officers had rotated through the organization. The nursing division was experiencing an equal amount of transition. Tenured leaders were leaving and the organizational landscape was shifting. Among all of this change, the front-line staff remained focused on clinical care. Their focus on practice and clinical excellence was apparent. The clinical outcomes were typically in the upper quartile in publically reported databanks. However, the culture indicators were reflecting negative trends: voluntary nurse turnover rates increased 16% to 18% and nurse turnover during the first year of employment was more than 30%. Employee-, patient-, and physician-engagement scores ranked below the 50th percentile.

The culture had a palpable sense of fear and relief. Wolf Creek partners define fear and relief as a culture that reflects scarcity, self preservation, withdrawing, and silence. This culture is in contrast to a learn-and-serve culture that reflects courage, risk taking, creativity, and unlimited accountability.[13] As the executive team began to establish themselves in their roles, it was critical to quickly measure the culture. The executive team designed a full-day retreat. With more than 150 leaders present, each was given three different colored dots. Green dots represented learn-and-serve culture, red dots represented fear-and-relief culture, and yellow dots represented something in between. Each leader chose the colored dot that they believed indicated the current organizational culture. Eighty percent of the dots that were placed on the spectrum were red. Approximately 15% were yellow and 5% were green.

It was clear that cultural change needed to occur. Believing that change needs to occur at the top, the senior executive team completed a 360-degree assessment of their individual leadership strengths. The 360-degree assessment tool utilized was the Leadership Circle Profile. The Leadership Circle Profile is designed to integrate many of the best theoretical frameworks from leadership, adult development, psychological, and spiritual bodies of knowledge. The Leadership Circle Profile is designed to measure behavior and assumptions simultaneously. The top half of the circle is labeled "Creative" and the bottom half is labeled "Reactive." The top half of the circle contains an array of 18 "Creative Competencies." These are competencies that have been shown, through leadership research, to be highly correlated to effectiveness and business outcomes. The creative-leadership competencies measure key behaviors and internal assumptions that lead to high-fulfillment and high-achievement leadership. There are 18 creative competencies built into five dimensions. The reactive leadership styles reflect inner beliefs and assumptions that limit effectiveness, authentic expression, and empowering leadership. There are 11 competencies built into three dimensions (**Table 1**).

Each member of the senior team self selected a minimum of 10 people to complete their profile. In addition, their immediate supervisor was instructed to complete the profile. Everyone also completed a profile on themselves. Results were returned to an independent coach, who then reviewed the profile with each senior team member. A coach was hired to work with each executive. With their coach, each individual created an action plan specific to the individual profile. The coach would meet with the executive on a monthly basis to ensure that focus and leadership change was occurring.

One specific leadership profile depicted strong creative tendencies (**Fig. 1**). As the coach debriefed this leader, the coach learned that coaching had been part of her leadership development for almost a decade. Utilizing a coach bimonthly was the norm for this leader. She realized early in her career that she needed a coach to be

Table 1
Creative leadership competencies

Creative Dimension	Definition
Relating	Measures the leaders' interest in and ability to connect and relate to others in a way that brings out the best in people, groups, and organizations
Creative competencies:	
Caring connection	Measures the leader's interest in and ability to form warm, caring relationships
Foster team play	Measures the ability to foster high-performance teamwork
Collaborator	Measures the extent to which the leader engages others in a manner that allows the parties involved to discover common ground
Mentoring and developing	Measures the ability to foster growth and personal and professional development in others
Interpersonal intelligence	Measures the interpersonal effectiveness to listen, engage in conflict and controversy, deal with the feelings of others, and manage their own feelings
Creative dimension	
Self awareness	Measures the orientation to ongoing professional and personal development and the degree to which inner-self awareness is expressed through high-integrity leadership
Creative competencies:	
Selfless leader	Measures the extent to which the leader pursues service over self interest
Balance	Measures the ability, in the midst of conflicting tensions of modern life, to keep a hearty balance between family and business, activity and reflection, work and leisure
Composure	Measures the ability, in the midst of conflict and high-tension situations, to remain composed and centered and to maintain a calm, focused perspective
Personal learner	Measures the degree to which the leader demonstrates a strong and active interest in learning, personal, and professional growth
Creative dimension	
Authenticity	Measures the capability to relate to others in an authentic, courageous, and high-integrity manner
Creative competency	
Integrity	Measures how well a leader adheres to the set of values and principles that you espouse
Courageous authenticity	Measures the willingness to take tough stands, bring up topics that are not discussable

Dimension	
Systems awareness	Measures the degree to which the leader's awareness is focused on whole-system improvement and on community welfare
Creative competency	
Community concern	Measures the service orientation from which the leader leads and the extent to which the leader links their legacy to service of community and global welfare
Sustainable productivity	Measures the ability to achieve results in a way that maintains or enhances the overall long-term effectiveness of the organization
Systems thinker	Measures the degree to which the leader thinks and acts from a whole-system perspective and the extent to which the leader makes decisions in light of the long-term health of the whole system
Dimension	
Achieving	Measures the extent to which the leader offers visionary, authentic, and high-achievement leadership
Creative competency	
Strategic focus	Measures the extent to which the leader thinks and plans rigorously and strategically to ensure that the organization will thrive in the near and long-term
Purposeful and visionary	Measures the extent to which the leader clearly communicates and models commitment to personal purpose and organizational vision
Achieves results	Measures the degrees to which the leader is goal directed and has a track record of goal achievement and high performance
Decisiveness	Measures the ability to make decisions on time and the extent to which the leader is comfortable moving forward in uncertainty
Reactive dimension	
Controlling	Measures the extent to which the leader establishes a sense of personal worth through task accomplishment and personal achievement
Reactive competency	
Perfect	Measures the leader's need to attain flawless results and perform to extremely high standards to feel secure and worthwhile as a person
Driven	Measures the extent to which the leader is in overdrive, and their belief that worth and security is tied to accomplishing a great deal through hard work, and their need to perform at a high level to feel worthwhile as a person

(continued on next page)

Table 1
(continued)

Creative Dimension	Definition
Ambition	Measures the extent to which the leader needs to get ahead, move up in the organization, and is better than others
Autocratic	Measures the tendency to be forceful, aggressive, and controlling, and the extent to which the leader equates self worth and security to being powerful, in control, strong, dominant, invulnerable, or on top. Worth is measured through comparison, that is having more income, achieving a higher position, being seen as a most/more valuable contributor, gaining credit, or being promoted
Reactive dimension	
Protecting	Measures the belief that the leader can protect themselves and establish a sense of worth through withdrawal, remaining distant, hidden, aloof, cynical, superior, or rational
Reactive competency	
Arrogance	Measures the tendency to project a large ego behavior that is experienced as superior, egotistical, and self centered
Critical	Measures the tendency to take a critical, questioning, and somewhat cynical attitude
Distance	Measures the tendency to establish a sense of personal worth and security through withdrawal, being superior, remaining aloof, emotionally distant, and above it all
Reactive dimension	
Complying	Measures the extent to which the leader gets a sense of self worth and security by complying with the expectations of others rather than acting on intent and want
Reactive competency	
Conservative	Measures the extent to which the leader thinks and acts conservatively, follows procedure, and lives within the prescribed rules of the organization
Pleasing	Measures the need to seek others' support and approval to feel secure and worthwhile as a person
Belonging	Measures the need to conform, follow the rules, and meet the expectation of those in authority
Passive	Measures the degree to which the leader gives away their power to others and to circumstances outside their control

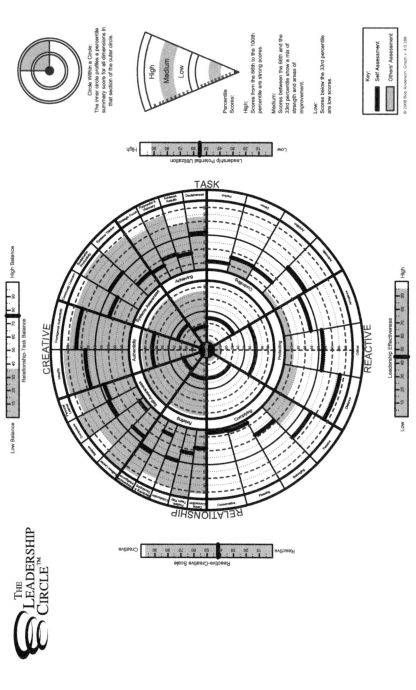

Fig. 1. The Leadership Circle Profile of individual leader. (Courtesy of Leadership Circle LLC; with permission.)

effective. The comparison she made was similar to how people utilize personal trainers. Just like personal trainers assist people in adhering to their fitness plans, this leader believed that her professional coach ensured that she stayed true to her values. Her coach provided just-in-time feedback that provided a reflective, neutral colleague who could assist and guide her through leadership-development moments. Coaching was critical to her leadership success. Her professional accomplishments included achieving Magnet designation, numerous quality awards, and active involvement in working within a Malcolm Baldridge setting. This individual's profile demonstrates that when leaders lead with creative tendencies, the business results follow.

An aggregate profile of the senior team was also shared. The senior team also developed a team action plan. The creative tendency of balance was extremely low. The team agreed to work collectively on this tendency.

The executive team then brought the 360-degree profile assessment to the director team. The director and executive team followed the identical process. Each of the directors received their profile and an individual coach. Action-plan development, monthly coaching, and ongoing feedback were provided to ensure progress.

The organization also took the individual profiles and created an aggregate leadership profile. This profile was the aggregate results from the senior team and the director team (**Fig. 2**). The entire leadership team created an action plan based on this profile. Creating a caring connection was the core competency that needed development among the entire team.

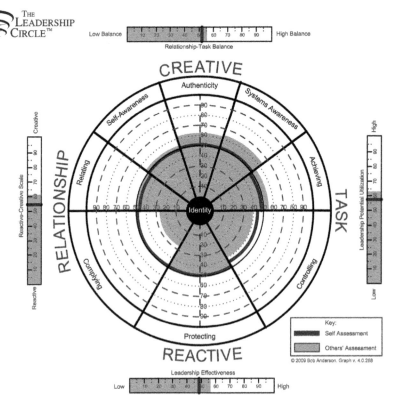

Fig. 2. A visual picture of an aggregate leadership profile. (*Courtesy of* Leadership Circle LLC; with permission.)

After almost 2 years of coaching, culture and business results demonstrated a positive direction. Over the 2 years, voluntary turnover ranged from 10% to 12%. Patient-satisfaction results were near the 75th percentile. Overall employee-engagement results improved to the 65th percentile. Prior to coaching, turnover rate was 18% and patient-satisfaction and employee-engagement results were below the 50th percentile. Based on these results, noticeable change occurred at the organizational level.

One specific leader chose to provide coaching to all of the formal leaders within her span of control. Shift coordinators, nurse managers, and the director received coaching. Her specific departmental results exceeded the organizational expectations. Patient satisfaction and employee satisfaction were in the top 10th percentile ranking within the organization. Clinical outcomes remained strong and operational metrics were significantly improved. Innovation and imagination were sparked. The critical-care unit implemented a closed-staffing model and their employee turnover and number of diversion hours dramatically declined. The short-stay telemetry unit developed a "Best in the Universe" retreat, where each staff member attended a full-day retreat. The focus of the retreat was on how, as a team, they could collectively rekindle the art of nursing. This specific team emulated positive deviant behavior and their overall outcomes were unmatched. Top box scores have been achieved in turnover rate, patient satisfaction, employee engagement, and physician satisfaction for this specific area.

SUMMARY

Based on this case study, it is clear that coaching can be an effective leadership intervention. Coaching should not be reserved for senior executives. The outcomes of this study identify that the coaching intervention was successful at all levels of leadership.

As organizations contemplate the use of coaching, introducing a 360-degree leadership-assessment tool is critical. Understanding the individual leadership tendencies allowed this organization to focus specifically on the behavior changes that were needed to move their leaders toward creative competencies. In addition to understanding the individual leadership tendencies, having an aggregate picture of how the leadership was leading proved insightful. The natural tendencies within this organization at the senior-team level and the director level were reactive. It was not surprising that because of this reactive culture, the organization experienced high turnover and low employee, patient, and physician engagement. This case study also demonstrates how leaders tend to mirror what they see. For example, the senior-team profile was a mirror image of the director profile. The senior team needed to set the example of creative leadership, so that the directors could emulate this new way of leading. Understanding the new leadership competencies was critical to start the cultural transformation.

Through effective use of coaches and clear communication to the leadership team regarding what competencies are needed to create success, the culture is slowly changing. The creative tendencies are gradually emerging. As health-care organizations continue to address the current challenges, offering coaching to the leadership team can help rebuild and re-energize cultures.

FURTHER IMPLICATIONS

Leaders need to create cultures that allow employees to thrive, not just survive. Further studies are needed that measure the impact reactive leaders have on an organization and contrast the impact that creative leaders have on a culture.

In addition, further validation of the coaching-effectiveness tool is needed. Organizations that invest in coaching might consider implementation of this tool to measure the effectiveness of this leadership intervention. Qualitative and quantitative results are necessary so that organizations can see the tangible difference coaching can have on the business.

REFERENCES

1. Anderson J. The leadership circle. Available at: www.leadershipcircle.com. Accessed August 12, 2009.
2. Secretan L. Reclaiming higher ground: creating organizations that inspire the soul. New York: Wiley, John, and Sons; 1997.
3. Hamel G. Moon shots for management. Harv Bus Rev 2009. February. p. 5.
4. Koloroutis M. Relationship-based care. Minneapolis (MN): Creative Health Care Management, Inc; 2004. p. 32–4.
5. Block P. The end of leadership, leader to leader. San Francisco, CA: Jossey-Bass Inc; 1997.
6. Wales S. Why coaching? J Change Manag 2002;2(2):275–82.
7. Weber PJ. Inspirational chaos: executive coaching and tolerance of complexity. 2005.
8. Ledgerwood G. From strategic planning to strategic coaching: evolving conceptual frameworks to enable changing business cultures. Participation and Empowerment: An International Journal 2003;1(1):46–56.
9. Lenhardt V. Coaching for meaning: the culture and practice of coaching and team building. New York: Palgrave; 2004.
10. Olivero G, Bane KD, Kopelman RE. Executive coaching as a transfer of training tool: effects on productivity in a public agency. Public Pers Manage 1997;26:4.
11. Thach EC. The impact of executive coaching and 360 feedback on leadership effectiveness. Leader Organ Dev J 2002;23:3–4.
12. Laske O. Can evidence-based coaching increase ROI. Participation and Empowerment: An International Journal 2004;2:2.
13. Available at: www.wolfcreekpartners.com. 2003. Accessed August 12, 2009.

Transformational Leadership: Application of Magnet's New Empiric Outcomes

Erin K. Meredith, ARNP-BC, PCCN[a],*, Elaine Cohen, RN, EdD, FAAN[a],
Lucille V. Raia, RN, MS, ARNP-BC, NEA-BC[b]

KEYWORDS

• Magnet • Transformation leadership • Empiric outcomes

The many benefits to hospitals throughout the world that achieved Magnet designation is well documented.[1–9] This status of recognition demands the support of leadership during the Magnet journey. In 2008, the American Nurses Credentialing Center (ANCC) announced a new model for the Magnet Recognition Program that translates the original 14 Forces of Magnetism into Five Model Components.[10] Specifically, this new model includes sources of evidence and empiric outcomes that by definition accentuates transformational nursing leadership. The day-to-day impact of this change places an even greater emphasis on demonstrated outcomes and innovation that may potentially transform nursing practice, quality and safety of care, and the population served. This article provides tangible examples and outcomes for reaching nursing excellence through leadership support and engagement.

TRANSFORMATIONAL LEADERSHIP

The transformational leadership component of the new Magnet Model is comprised of three categories:

• Strategic planning
• Advocacy and influence
• Visibility, accessibility, and communication.

---

[a] James A. Haley Veterans' Hospital, 13000 Bruce B. Downs Boulevard, Tampa, FL 33612, USA
[b] Nursing Education, James A. Haley Veterans' Hospital, 13000 Bruce B. Downs Boulevard, Tampa, FL 33612, USA
* Corresponding author.
E-mail address: erin.meredith@va.gov (E.K. Meredith).

Nurs Clin N Am 45 (2010) 49–64
doi:10.1016/j.cnur.2009.10.007   nursing.theclinics.com
0029-6465/10/$ – see front matter. Published by Elsevier Inc.

Each category is as valuable as the next in identifying and measuring leadership outcomes. A summary of the empiric outcomes for the transformational leadership component is illustrated in **Box 1**.

Strategic Planning Empiric Outcomes: Driving Forces

Specific outcomes are needed to demonstrate the effectiveness and efficiency of nursing's strategic planning. Certainly this cannot be accomplished with one strategic plan. One means to achieving and sustaining desired outcomes is by implementing interdisciplinary, evidence-based practice methods. As disciplines do not work in a vacuum, buy in, ownership, and the development of new processes must be designed to cross organizational service boundaries and include all team members.

The foundation for evidence-based practice (EBP) is well defined and encouraged. However, the role of leadership in evidence-based practice is less delineated. One of the first attempts to bridge this knowledge and application gap in nursing is Porter-O'Grady and Malloch's[11,12] work on quantum leadership. Their premise lies in the fact that the 21st century warrants more distinctive and unique leadership approaches than those used in past decades. The transition from the Industrial Age of the last century to the present Age of Technology has challenged health care organizations, insurers, and governments alike. The frameworks by which organizations were based today have morphed into designs that display linkages that are relational, dynamic, and fluid.[12] As Porter-O' Grady and Malloch so aptly state, "leaders therefore will be tasked with understanding and integrating the elements of change into new realities that are fast-moving, non-linear, and socially transformational." So to be successful, the nurse executive must communicate the vision of the organization, nursing's role, the effect on cost and quality of care, and professional and community implications.[13,14]

The concepts of efficiency and effectiveness are the outcomes by which organizations thrive and sustain. Accordingly, how do these concepts make a difference to the hallmark tenets of health care systems: cost, access, quality, and satisfaction? Porter-O'Grady and Malloch,[12] and others,[15–18] posit that health care systems are seeking answers to making a difference in patient outcomes, creating value-added care, preserving quality, and increasing access, while controlling cost. Wakefield[16] further argues that nursing can become a pivotal force in changing the existing structures of health care in the United States and Porter-O'Grady and Malloch,[12] speak to dismantling and transforming these structures to "reflect new relationships of workers

---

Box 1
Transformational leadership empiric outcomes

Strategic planning

The outcomes that result from strategic planning structures and processes used by nursing to improve the health care system's effectiveness and efficiency

Advocacy and influence

One Chief Nursing Officer-influenced organization-wide change

Visibility, accessibility, and communication

Changes in the work environment and patients' care based on input from the direct-care nurses

Courtesy of American Nurses Credentialing Center. Magnet recognition program: application manual. Silver Spring (MD); 2008; with permission.

with the purpose of their work in an environment of seamless, continuous, integration."

Application

Realizing these concepts would be our guiding principles, the nursing leadership team at the James A. Haley VA Hospital (JAHVH), a Magnet-designated organization since 2001, sought to develop an innovative and sustainable strategic plan based upon the tenets of quantum leadership. We began the journey of applying the principles of evidence-based leadership to meet the demands of our particular dynamic health care delivery system. Additionally, the strategic plan was aligned with the Magnet criteria; thus providing a fabric of diverse yet blended ideologies to guide the retreat. At the beginning of the Nursing Service Strategic Planning Retreat, a crosswalk was presented tying together the quantum-leadership categories, the previous year's Nursing Service Strategic Plan, the Hospitals' Strategic Plan, the 14 Forces of Magnetism, and the new Magnet Model components (**Table 1**).

Diverse groups, which included staff nurses, worked on the five quantum-leadership categories resulting in the final Nursing Service Strategic Plan (**Box 2**) that provides the opportunity for measuring the efficiency and effectiveness of our processes. Once a strategic plan is in place, leadership must be vigilant in holding the teams accountable, monitoring results of groups, and tracking outcomes.

Advocacy and Influence Empiric Outcome: Driving Forces

With nursing staff shortages and sicker patients with longer lengths of stay resulting in high bed occupancy, some hospitals are having difficulty with patient flow and longer-than-anticipated emergency room wait times. The JAHVH is no exception to these phenomena. The Associate Director (AD) and the Patient Care/Nursing Services (CNO) spearheaded a significant system-level performance-improvement change to provide timely and appropriate access to health care by implementing best practices.

The JAHVH begins every day with a bed occupancy of 94% in acute care and 97% in the ICUs. Patient throughput is an ongoing challenge that the AD monitors on a daily basis. In collaboration with the Chief Nurse of Acute Care, the AD implemented the principles of system redesign (formerly Advanced Clinic Access [ACA]) in the inpatient setting. Initially, Advanced Clinic Access was the veterans' affairs (VA) practice initiative in collaboration with Institute for Healthcare Improvement in ambulatory care settings to improve access to timely and efficient care. ACA was one method of putting VA philosophy of patient-centered care into practice. ACA thinking and concepts are now termed system redesign and uses many of the same principles from ACA:

- Shape the demand
  - Work down the backlog
  - Reduce demand
- Match supply and demand
  - Understand supply and demand
  - Reduce appointment types
  - Plan for contingencies
- Redesign the system to increase supply
  - Manage the constraint
  - Optimize the care team
  - Synchronize patients, provider, and information
  - Predict and anticipate patients' needs at time of appointment
  - Optimize rooms and equipment.

Table 1
2009 James A. Haley VA Hospital nursing service strategic planning retreat: reality crosswalk

Major Categories/ Quantum Leadership	Nursing Strategic Goals and Key Priorities 2007–2008	JAHVH and Clinics Strategic Plan 2008–2009	14 Forces of Magnetism	Five Magnet Model Components (New)
Physical environment	**Continuum of care** Polytrauma programs Advanced clinic access Emergency planning Survey readiness **Organizational excellence** Systems redesign and patient flow Safe, high reliability systems New directives and capacity for new requirements	**Access** Maximize use of space. Coordinate the delivery of services to maximize patient flow	Organizational structure (#2) Quality of care (patient safety [#7])	Structural empowerment Empiric quality outcomes Exemplary professional practice
Caregiver teams	**Continuum of care** Clinical nurse leader program **Employer of choice** Workforce development Mentoring and coaching programs High employee satisfaction	**Cost effectiveness** Optimize revenue generation Optimize VERA **Quality** Maintenance of maximal physical, mental, social, and spiritual function By 2009, involved in 12 community outreach events each year	Autonomy (#9) Quality of care(ethics, patient safety, and quality infrastructure [#7]) Interdisciplinary relationships (#13) Nurses as teachers (#11)	Exemplary professional practice Empiric quality outcomes New knowledge, innovations, and improvements

Patient care delivery model	**Continuum of care** Polytrauma programs Self-management programs (chronic disease, MOVE program) Case management(opioid chronic pain, HIV risk assessment) Community health **Evidenced-based decision making** Evidenced-based practice models Theoretical/conceptual models Research translation **Organizational excellence** Transforming Care at the Bedside (TCAB) **Excellence in customer service** Patient-centeredness model of care	**Cost effectiveness** Efficient use of resources **Quality** Create a safe patient environment in all health-care settings Maximize physical, mental, social, and spiritual function facility-wide Restoration of function across the board Optimize the health of the veterans in VA community and contribute to the health of nation	Professional models of care (#5) Consultation & resources (#8) Autonomy (#9) Organizational structure (#2) Community and health care organization (#10)	Exemplary professional practice Empiric quality outcomes New knowledge, innovations, and improvements
Technology	**Evidence-based decision making** Technology innovations **Continuum of care** Technology(telehealth initiatives, My Health e-Vet, electronic tools) **Employer of choice** Streamlined administrative processes affecting personnel **Organizational excellence** Initiatives to improve clinical outcomes Performance measures and monitors Unit-based performance improvement	**Access** Create process for tracking, forecasting, planning, and modeling demand for services	Quality improvement (#7) Quality of care (research and evidenced-based practice [#6])	Structural empowerment Empiric quality outcomes New knowledge, innovations, and improvements

(continued on next page)

Table 1
(continued)

Major Categories/ Quantum Leadership	Nursing Strategic Goals and Key Priorities 2007–2008	JAHVH and Clinics Strategic Plan 2008–2009	14 Forces of Magnetism	Five Magnet Model Components (New)
Culture	**Continuum of care** New patient orientation and enrollment **Excellence in customer service** Excellence in patient satisfaction Shared decision making model Internal customer satisfaction **Employer of choice** Leadership development Shared governance structure for professional practice Safe environment for staff and patients Separation of Tampa and Orlando	**Satisfaction** Become employer of choice by 2010. Promote staff development Establish an integrated and synergistic learning environment for all staff. Improve overall patient satisfaction and patient-centered care. Restructure and empower customer service council for PI. **Quality** Veterans, employees, and community recognize JAHVH as the leader in health care quality	Quality of nursing leadership (#1) Management style (#3) Image of nursing (#12) Professional development (#14) Personnel policies and programs (#4) Organizational structure (#7)	Transformational leadership Structural empowerment Exemplary professional practice New knowledge, innovations, and improvements

Abbreviations: MOVE, managing overweight and/or obesity for veterans everywhere; PI, performance improvement; VERA, veterans' equitable resource allocation.

Box 2
JAHVH nursing service strategic plan 2009–2011

1. Physical environment

A healing environment sustains competent care providers, increases patient/staff satisfaction and safety, and minimizes adverse outcomes.

Goal #1: Enhance patient comfort at the unit-based level (Knowledge Worker [KW]).

Goal #2: Enhance patient comfort measures hospital wide (Leaders [L]).

Goal #3: Promote unit-specific monitoring of safety issues (Managers [M]).

Goal #4: Enhance hospital-wide infection control measures (KW, M, L).

Goal #5: Address noise-reduction issues (KW, M, L).

Goal #6: Restructure environment-of-care rounds to reflect the link between auxiliary patient care and point-of-care services (KW, M, L).

2. Caregiver teams

Availability of healthy, engaged, and productive staff positively impacts program and facility goals (the right caregivers, doing the right thing, at the right time).

Goal #1: Improve seamless communication and interaction among all services to reduce duplication and effort (ie, hand off; [KW]).

Goal #2: Improve "unit perceived quality of care" (NDNQI) through staff accountability and responsibility for overall patient-care quality (KW).

Goal #3: Promote interdisciplinary teamwork and interpersonal skills among all services to include a respectful and nurturing environment (KW, M, L).

Goal #4: Assure the application of evidence-based practice as defined and developed by clinical experts (ie, heart failure, polytrauma; [KW, M, L]).

3. Patient-care delivery models

Successful patient-care delivery systems are those where care is organized and delivered to promote seamless, evidence-based interventions in a timely manner.

Goal #1: Increase specialty certifications 25% by 2015 (KW).

Goal #2: Increase overall BSN Workforce 25% by 2020 (KW).

Goal #3: Ensure continuity and coordination of care by decreasing the redundancy and duplication of nursing documentation in CPRS (KW, M, L).

Goal #4: Increase access to support services and equipment availability throughout facility (KW, M, L).

Goal #5: Full implementation of the clinical nurse leaders and patient care facilitator roles (M, L).

4. Technology

Decisions to invest in technology must be value enhancing for patients, caregivers, and the organization.

Goal #1: Implement computerized self scheduling for nursing staff (KW, M).

Goal #2: Expand usage of care-management dashboard to nursing and all providers (KW, M).

Goal #3: Assess technical competence/usage in the veteran population (KW, M, L).

5. Culture

Build an organizational infrastructure that supports innovation, dissemination of information, care transformation, value- and evidence-based decision making, and long-term sustainability.

> **Goal #1:** Promote creative scheduling to support staff in their educational endeavors and career advancements (KW, M).
>
> **Goal #2:** Implement an evidence-based leadership model and articulate the three key roles of knowledge worker, manager, and leader (KW, M, L).
>
> - Nurses will have a comprehensive understanding of their roles
> - Application of their role with patients, families, communities, and the interdisciplinary team
> - Application of new knowledge and evidence (ie, Transforming Care at the Bedside [TCAB])
>
> *Abbreviations:* BSN, bechelor of science in nursing; CPRs, computerized patient record system; NDNQI, national database of nursing quality indicators.

ACA/system redesign principles were implemented in the inpatient setting and as a result the following changes were made:

- Morning labs are drawn earlier to facilitate early patient discharge.
- Development of Nursing Officers of the Day position to assist with bed placement.
- Bed Management System was implemented using a color-coded, visual, easy-to-access, inpatient census program that interfaces with VISTA computer software.
- Monthly interdisciplinary hospital patient flow meetings were started.
- An admissions nurse position was implemented in the emergency department (ED) for faster admission to the units.
- A daily veterans' integrated service network 8 bed huddle call to identify bed vacancies within our region was started. (Inpatient mental health beds at the JAHVH are at a premium.)
- More telemetry and ICU beds were added.
- A physician telemetry protocol was developed, along with a memorandum of understanding between the ED and the Chief of Medicine to reduce unnecessary bed movement.
- Pharmacy runners were added to assist with patient discharges.
- The discharge appointment monitor was fully met.
- There was a tightening of use-management (UM) oversight, resulting in increased appropriateness of admissions.
- Anticipated discharge orders and appointments were implemented.
- Home intravenous antibiotics were outsourced.
- Hospice referrals were reorganized.
- Inpatients needing hemodialysis are discharged before their treatment.
- Plan, Do, Study, Act is performed to address isolation and private rooms in response to the methicillin-resistant staphylococcus aureus (MRSA) directive. On the medical, surgical, and telemetry units, four four-bed rooms have been dedicated for colonized patients who have MRSA.
- The operating room (OR) hired a full-time scheduler, focusing on elective surgeries.
- Internal OR flow meetings are held to improve OR efficiency.
- A transportation workgroup was established, including volunteers to drive patients to and from the facility for appointments.
- Patient care facilitator positions were created to assist with patient discharge.
- Bed-cleaning turnaround has been increased.

Improving the appropriateness of admissions also benefits the flow of patients. By ensuring that patients who do not meet full admission criteria are admitted under a 23-hour observation assists in rapid discharge, if appropriate for patients. Education with providers and monitoring by UM nurses have improved our discharge process. In addition, the AD monitors the number of 23-hour admissions during daily staffing meetings.

Changing the way physicians round on their patients has also resulted in increased bed availability in the ED, ICUs, and medical-surgical units. Traditionally, patients were pushed through the system where physicians round on patients in the ICUs first and then go to the medical-surgical units. As demand for beds increased in the ED, patients were forced out or patients waited for hours in the ED. Now, physicians begin rounds on the telemetry units where patients can be discharged. Stable ICU patients can be moved out of their units to make room for ED patients. Time between cases has decreased because of the efforts of the OR. There has also been a reduction in first case start delays. The JAHVH received a Certificate of Appreciation from the Southeast Regional Flow Improvement Collaborative in recognition of our pioneering work to improve inpatient flow.

Visibility, Accessibility, and Communication Empiric Outcomes: Driving Forces

Magnet organization leaders are constantly listening to their employees for ways to improve the work environment and patients' care. The best people to ask are those intimately involved, the direct care nurses. Another hallmark of a Magnet organization is to have several mechanisms in place for staff to provide input. At the JAHVH, these mechanisms include hospital town hall meetings; staff participation in root cause analysis; hospital committees, such as safety and CPR, performance improvement teams, product evaluations, and construction/expansion projects; and implementing a culture that fosters shared decision making and evidence-based practice.

Table 2
United States Preventive Services Task Force strength-of-evidence rating and the Agency for Healthcare Research and Quality evidence hierarchy scales

Level I	Meta-analysis (combination of data from many studies)
Level II	Experimental designs (randomized control trials)
Level III	Well-designed, quasi-experimental designs (not randomized or no control group)
Level IV	Well-designed, non-experimental designs (descriptive, can include qualitative)
Level V	Case reports/clinical expertise
Strength of evidence	
United States Preventive Services Task Force grading	
A	Strongly recommended; good evidence
B	Recommended; at least fair evidence
C	No recommendation; balance of benefits and harms too close to justify a recommendation
D	Recommend against; fair evidence is ineffective or harm outweighs the benefit
E	Insufficient evidence; evidence is lacking or of poor quality, benefit and harms cannot be determined

Data from US Preventive Services Task Force. Guide to clinical preventive services. 2nd edition. Washington, DC: Office of Disease Prevention and Health Promotion; 1996; Agency for Healthcare Research and Quality. Systems to rate the strength of scientific evidence. Fact sheet. AHRQ Publication No. 02–P0022, Rockville (MD): Agency for Healthcare Research and Quality; 2002. Available at: http://www.ahrq.gov/clinic/epcsums/strenfact.htm. Accessed July 10, 2009.

Table 3
Transforming care at the bedside innovations at James A. Haley VA Hospital

Ideas from Kick Off	Safety/Reliability	Workforce Vitality	Patient Centered	Efficiency (Lean)
Need weight scales that do not break down	—	New beds have a built-in scale	—	—
If no nurse is at the nurses' station, call lights do not get a timely answer. Most calls are for morning care items.	Unit clerk trained to answer call lights	—	Utility carts ordered for items frequently asked for	—
Help physicians know which nurse is making rounds with them	—	—	—	Posting daily roster of nurse assigned to make rounds on each physician team and which nurse is assigned to patients about to be discharged
Need immediate feedback after adverse events or other changes in environment	Safety huddle after any adverse event or near miss and also an update huddle; data posted for staff	—	—	—
Reduce noise and improve communication (nurse-to-nurse, nurse-to-physician, and nurse-to-SPD)	—	—	—	Implemented Vocera (hands-free communication device)
Reduce possible cross-contamination of computers on wheels in isolation rooms	Develop procedure for scanning medications in isolation rooms, and for flocart cleaning	—	—	—
Clarification of role of the volunteers with SCI patients	Guidelines developed for volunteers so patients can stay on diet and fluid restriction and be safely fed	—	—	—

Issue / Opportunity	Action taken
Lost patient belongings	Receipt book for patient belongings; Added question to discharge note as reminder to take home belongings
More secure and less obtrusive method to secure laboratory specimens before delivery to laboratory	Have a mailbox with red flag for "Please pick up," which is nicer looking and protects specimens
Cancelled surgeries among same-day admissions and delays among inpatient surgeries	Recommendations made to reduce missed or late laboratory draws, type, and cross
Patients were too passive about their medications	List of each day's medications are distributed to patients at 7AM
Patients are coffee drinkers and it is only served at breakfast	Food service delivers each day an extra large container of coffee, stirrers, sugar, sugar substitute, creamers, etc
Nursing is not systematically included in rounds	Nurse on rounds with each attending team
Establish method to increase accountability for activities assigned	Accountability/responsibility form implemented
Not enough time to set goals and plans before starting 9AM medications	Pharmacy changed times from 9-1-5 to 10-2-6
Communicating non-urgent information to physicians	"Dear Doctor" forms for nurses or families to use to leave at bedside for rounds

(continued on next page)

Table 3
(continued)

Ideas from Kick Off	Safety/Reliability	Workforce Vitality	Patient Centered	Efficiency (Lean)
Help when patients are in pre-code status	Medical response team established throughout campus	—	—	—
Most admissions are in evenings and often after food service is closed	—	—	In addition to box lunches, frozen meals are now provided as another alternative	—
Patients do not have individual TVs in multi-bed rooms	—	—	Wall installation completed for over-bed TVs	—
Patients need reassurance that staff are available	Nurses now park computer on wheels in four-bed rooms for better access to patients	—	Comfort and safety rounds every 2 hours; list developed of items to offer patients (toilet, refreshments, etc)	—
Delays in discharge are occurring because of minor things overlooked	—	—	—	Discharge checklist accompanies each rounds team
In present configuration, nurses have to run to a front desk for pages, delaying response time	—	—	—	Phone lines installed in back halls and side halls
Running out of medications in frequent use	—	New stock levels established for Pyxis	—	—
Location of whiteboards is not ergonomically correct	—	—	Consultation obtained to determine ergonomically correct placement	—
Poorly designed nurses locker room	—	Redesigned and made more usable	—	—

Family assessment skill training	—	—	Prepares for reintegration into the community	—	—
Volunteer as patient feeders; guidelines developed	—	—	Faster service at lunch time	—	Incentive developed for more volunteers
Reduce hunting and gathering time	—	—	—	—	Combine medication room and supply room
White boards for goals and plans, discharge date, nurse's name, notes for doctor	—	—	Incorporates patient into planning for care, and progress toward mutual goals	—	—
Transporters for evening; desired for night, combining with runner	—	—	—	—	Implemented with temporary workers without compensation
Text messaging of physicians for non-urgent things	—	—	—	—	Saves phone-tag time
Patient packet to orient to unit	—	—	Also useful for families	—	—
Formal tests of patient readiness for discharge	—	—	—	—	To improve patient flow
Palliative care consults	—	—	Physician-led team established; education begun	—	—
Post code reviews	Tested on telemetry unit	—	—	—	—
Developing RN care pathways for thoracic surgery	—	—	Provides markers of progress	—	—
Developed thoracic surgery physician order sets	Avoid communication gaps	—	—	—	—
New lighting in patient rooms for visibility and safety	Good response from patients	—	—	—	—
Additional frozen meals for patients admitted on evenings and weekends	—	—	Better than wrapped sandwiches with little choice	—	—

(continued on next page)

Table 3
(continued)

Ideas from Kick Off	Safety/Reliability	Workforce Vitality	Patient Centered	Efficiency (Lean)
Admission/discharge nurse when staffing allows	—	Some discharge duties assumed by RN patient care facilitators	—	—
20-ft ambulation markers established on baseboards	—	—	Helps patients to independently measure ambulation ability	—
Patient shower shoes (shared showers on units)	—	—	Appropriate and considerate	—
Safe patient handling equipment and devices	Implemented throughout inpatient areas and some areas like endoscopy, radiology, OR	—	—	—
Newsletter to enhance communication among unit staff	—	12-hour shifts mean many are only on unit 3 days per week	—	—
Charge nurse handoff	—	—	—	Although safety and vitality are also addressed, it is communication that is improved
Yakker trackers	—	—	Reducing noise is a goal	—
Staff recognition boards	—	To allow staff to reward one another for going the extra mile	—	—
Critical event simulation	Practice sessions for cardiac arrest and other emergencies	—	—	—

Abbreviations: RN, registered nurse; SCI, spinal cord injury; SPD, supply, processing and distribution.

Application
A powerful tool the JAHVH has implemented for staff to have a say over their practice is providing a foundation for evidence-based practice. Supported by the AD and led by the Nursing Research Committee, the adoption of an EBP model to serve as a guide for staff was crucial. After reviewing several models, the Iowa model was selected. In addition, to assist staff with the practice and application of EBP, the US Preventive Services Task Force Strength of Evidence rating[19] and the Agency for Healthcare Research and Quality evidence hierarchy scales[20] were adopted to grade evidence (**Table 2**). Nursing research workshops and Internet-based continuing education courses are also offered to the staff.

Another mechanism for incorporating EBP into daily practice is the development of an EBP Fellowship. The EBP Fellowship is a 3- to 6-month part-time position for a staff nurse to research a nursing service priority. Our current EBP fellow is researching interventions to reduce ventilator associated pneumonia rates in the ICUs. Other examples employed at the JAHVH to allow direct-care nurses control and input over their work environment and patient care is TCAB.[21] TCAB work has been so successful that it has been adopted by all of our acute-care inpatient units.

By respecting the opinions of staff nurses, many of our nursing teams have been inspired to participate in resolving issues and developing innovative approaches to patient care. Staff nurses have adopted professional-practice models that are best matched to their respective care delivery areas. Each acute-care unit that has rolled out the TCAB processes has individualized it to their specialty patient populations. TCAB allows direct-care nurses to identify performance improvement projects and perform rapid tests of change on these new ideas. The TCAB tenet of "patient-centered care" resulted in the use of white boards to enhance the communication process between patients, families, physician teams, nursing staff, and ancillary services. The use of white boards has subsequently spread throughout the hospital. In addressing two more TCAB tenets, "safety and reliability" and "vitality and team-work," direct-care nurses used the principles of "lean" to evaluate access and security of medications and supplies. The outcome resulted in a move toward establishing Pyxis supply centers on inpatient units and installing two profile Pyxis medication dispensing towers on larger nursing units to assure expedient, convenient, and safe medication administration. Other changes that have occurred because of TCAB are outlined in (**Table 3**).

SUMMARY

Porter-O'Grady and Malloch[11] exquisitely state that "evidence for leadership requires engaged reasoning and critical analysis that considers multiple sources of knowledge." Applying this understanding and infusing the work environment with transformational leadership builds an infrastructure of cultural innovation that will certainly outlive its originators. Many of the initiatives highlighted in this article were possible because of the innovative and open leadership style of our leadership team. Likewise, the engagement and futuristic thinking of the nursing staff has established a practice community that positions our entire organization to take full advantage of any change that is out in the health care horizon.

REFERENCES

1. Armstrong K, Laschinger H, Wong C. Workplace empowerment and magnet hospital characteristics as predictors of patient safety climate. J Nurs Care Qual 2009;24(1):55–62.

2. Stordeur S, D'Hoore W. Organizational configuration of hospitals succeeding in attracting and retaining nurses. J Adv Nurs 2007;57(1):45–58.
3. Kramer M, Schmalenberg C. Magnet hospitals: what makes nurses stay? Nursing 2004;34(6):50–4.
4. Kramer M, Schmalenberg C. Magnet hospital staff nurses describe clinical autonomy. Nurs Outlook 2003;51(1):13–9.
5. Laschinger HK, Almost J, Tuer-Hodes D. Workplace empowerment and magnet hospital characteristics: making the link. J Nurs Adm 2003;33(7–8):410–22.
6. Upenieks VV. The interrelationship of organizational characteristics of magnet hospitals, nursing leadership, and nursing job satisfaction. Health Care Manag 2003;22(2):83–98.
7. Upenieks VV. What constitutes effective leadership? Perceptions of magnet and nonmagnet nurse leaders. J Nurs Adm 2003;33(9):456–67.
8. Upenieks VV. Assessing differences in job satisfaction of nurses in magnet and nonmagnet hospitals. J Nurs Adm 2002;32(11):564–76.
9. Aiken LH, Smith HL, Lake ET. Lower Medicare mortality among a set of hospitals known for good nursing care. Med Care 1994;32(8):771–87.
10. American Nurses Credentialing Center. Magnet recognition program: application manual. Silver Spring (MD): American Nurses Credentialing Center; 2008.
11. Porter-O'Grady T, Malloch K. Beyond myth and magic: the future of evidence-based leadership. Nurs Adm Q 2008;32(3):176–87.
12. Porter-O'Grady T, Malloch K. Quantum leadership: a resource for health care innovation. 2nd edition. Boston: Jones and Bartlett; 2007.
13. Steinbinder A. Bumps on the road to magnet designation: achieving organizational excellence. Nurs Adm Q 2009;33(2):99–104.
14. Tagnesi K, Dumon C, Rawlinson C. The CNO: challenges and opportunities on the journey to excellence. Nurs Adm Q 2009;33(2):159–67.
15. Erwin D. Changing organizational performance: examining the change process. Hosp Top 2009;87(3):28–40.
16. Wakefield M. Envisioning and implementing new directions for health care. Nurs Econ 2008;26(1):49–51.
17. Vlasses F, Smeltzer C. Toward a new future for healthcare and nursing practice. J Nurs Adm 2007;17(9):375–80.
18. Titler MG, Kleiber C, Steelman VJ, et al. The Iowa model of evidence-based practice to promote quality care. Crit Care Nurs Clin North Am 2001;13(4):497–509.
19. U.S. Preventive Services Task Force. Guide to clinical preventive services. 2nd edition. Washington, DC: Office of Disease Prevention and Health Promotion; 1996.
20. Agency for Healthcare Research and Quality. Systems to rate the strength of scientific evidence. Rockville (MD): Agency for Healthcare Research and Quality; 2002. Fact sheet. AHRQ Publication No. 02–P0022. Available at: http://www.ahrq.gov/clinic/epcsums/strenfact.htm. Accessed July 10, 2009.
21. Institute for Healthcare Improvement. Innovation series: transforming care at the bedside. Cambridge (MA): IHI; 2004. Available at: http://www.rwjf.org/files/publications/other/IHITCABpaper[1].pdf. Accessed July 10, 2009.

The Effect of Telephone Nurse Triage on the Appropriate Use of the Emergency Department

Robert L. Dent, DNP, MBA, RN, NEA-BC, FACHE

KEYWORDS

• Emergency department • Telephone nurse triage
• ED throughput

In early 2008, the president of the Governing Board and another board member met with the Interim Director, Emergency Services and the Vice President/Chief Nursing Officer regarding the numbers of complaints received from patients visiting the emergency department at Midland Memorial Hospital. On reviewing the outcomes being achieved at the time, patient satisfaction was very low; more than 14% of patients who registered left without being seen by a medical provider, and the average time it took for a patient to see a medical provider after registration was more than 75 minutes. Wait times of up to 6 hours were being reported. The outcomes reported in this emergency department were similar to many being reported around the nation.

SETTING AND SIGNIFICANCE

Midland County has a total population of 123,532 (Bureau, US Census).[1] In a quality review of patients registered at the Midland Memorial Hospital (MMH) Emergency Department (ED) over a 10-month timeframe, October 2007 to August 2008 (n = 42,952), up to 61% of the patients treated could be considered inappropriate for care in an ED. The medical director of Emergency Services at MMH defined appropriate use of the ED as those patients coded in Tier 4 and Tier 5. Some patients in Tier 3 may be appropriate users of the ED if releasing them, or not treating them, may cause a more serious outcome than if treated in the emergency department (Wilson, 2008).[2,3] Patients visiting the emergency department coded as Tier 1 or Tier 2 patients are considered nonurgent or nonemergent, and may be inappropriate users of the emergency department.

Midland Memorial Hospital, Midland, 2200 West Illinois Avenue, TX 79701, USA
E-mail address: bob.dent@midland-memorial.com

Nurs Clin N Am 45 (2010) 65–69
doi:10.1016/j.cnur.2009.10.003   nursing.theclinics.com
0029-6465/10/$ – see front matter © 2010 Elsevier Inc. All rights reserved.

Implementing low-cost interventions, such as a telephone nurse triage (TNT) system, were needed to improve the appropriate use of the ED. The appropriate use of the ED, in turn, could improve revenue, patient satisfaction, and nurse/provider satisfaction.

REVIEW OF LITERATURE

A comprehensive review of the literature was completed, covering a 10-year period from 1999 to 2008, through electronic databases. The key words used were "ED triage," "nurse phone triage," and "decreasing ED visits."

There were 36 articles reviewed. Twenty-five articles were selected for the purpose of this literature review as there was enough evidence to make a decision to implement a TNT line. Three key themes emerged: reduction in inappropriate use of the ED, patient satisfaction, and a safe alternative. There were 7 articles highlighted.

REDUCTIONS IN INAPPROPRIATE USE OF EMERGENCY DEPARTMENT

Fortune and colleagues[4–6] completed a literature review of 36 articles over an 11-year period, 1989 to 2000, to investigate the benefits of recommended practices of implementing a TNT system. The findings showed up to a 73% reduction in the inappropriate use of the ED with the effective use of a TNT system.

Light and colleagues[7] conducted a descriptive correlation study of 110 nonrandom samples of parents who called the TNT line over a 2-year period. The study investigated whether home-care advice given by nurses changed parents' original preference for care. Eighty percent (80%) of these parents followed the advice of the nurse for home care, and 72% of parents whose original inclination was to take their child to the ED or physician's office accepted the nurse's advice for home care. The researchers concluded the TNT reduces unnecessary visits to the ED or physician's office and saves money, time, and emotional trauma.

These 2 articles illustrate that TNTs can reduce the inappropriate use of the ED.

PATIENT SATISFACTION

Cariello and colleagues[8–10] surveyed 300 randomly selected callers using a modified version of the SERVQUAL tool. The survey was administered by telephone during a 1-week period in 1999 to study the service quality from the perception of the callers who used a TNT system on behalf of pediatric patients. Those surveyed rated the quality of service as 6.42 of a possible 7.0, and 99% of callers indicated they would use this service again. Cariello[8] was able to quantify a 36.8% reduction in costs derived from the difference in original inclination and change in disposition with TNT.

Greenberg[11] surveyed 90 clients who had recently experienced the TNT system in a descriptive study during a 1-month period. The findings showed 91% of callers agreed with the nurses' suggestions, 88% followed the nurses' instructions, and the level of satisfaction was 8.2 (SD = 1.5) on a scale of 9 (89% of callers responded with an 8 or 9). This researcher too was able to quantify a cost savings for the service.

Hagan and colleagues[12,13] surveyed 4696 callers to the TNT line from October 6, 1997 to December 15, 1997. The findings showed more than 94% of callers were satisfied, 84% of callers considered the recommendations effective, 95% of callers considered the call useful in solving problems, 92.5% of callers would use the service again, and 80% of respondents felt they saved 5 hours of their time.

These 3 articles reported increases in patient satisfaction.

SAFE ALTERNATIVE

Dale and colleagues[14–16] collected data as part of a pragmatic randomized controlled trial study reported elsewhere. A panel reviewed 231 sets of case notes to assess the safety of nurses offering telephone triage as an alternative to emergency dispatch for nonurgent patients. The majority of the panel agreed with the decisions in 96.7% of the cases that emergency dispatch and care was not needed, and concluded that TNT is a safe alternative with no evidence that safety had been compromised.

Larson-Dahn[17] reviewed 10 consecutive TNT cases for 5 nurses in a quality assurance procedure review of documentation. The findings showed statistically significant relationships between disposition and critical thinking ($r = -0.374$; $P<.01$), disposition rating and continuity of care ($r = 0.296$; $P<.05$), assessment and critical thinking ($r = 0.479$; $P<.01$), and health outcomes and advice being followed ($r = 0.660$; $P<.01$). The findings show it is possible that following the advice of the telephone triage nurse improved health outcomes.

These 2 articles indicate that for many conditions, TNT is a safe alternative to ED visits that are inappropriate.

REQUIREMENTS FOR IMPLEMENTATION AND SUSTAINABILITY

The success of a TNT line is dependent on the acceptance of TNT by the community as an adequate source for receiving triage advice to the most appropriate place to receive care. Equally important is assuring funding and administrative, physician, and board support. Sustainability of a TNT line includes the ongoing support of the service. In today's cost-effective focused society, a TNT line must show a benefit to the residents and to the organization through better use of emergency services, as evidenced by more appropriate use of the ED and improved income through a reduction in bad debt.

DISCUSSION

Whereas a TNT service may be adequate to appropriately place patients, patients may be referred to the ED due to limited access to primary care and clinic appointments.[18–26] Thus, there are other issues to the overcrowding and inappropriate use of the ED that need to be addressed, including access to primary care providers and community clinics.[19,20,23,27] If there is inadequate access to either of these entities, the ED will continue to see those patients considered inappropriate.

In conclusion, the results of this review indicate that the use of a TNT is likely to be a safe method for triaging patients to the most appropriate place to receive care. Further, the TNT services may improve the appropriate use of the ED.

After several weeks of intense marketing, a phone number, managed 24 hours per day, was implemented July 6, 2009, for the purposes of receiving calls and triaging persons to the most appropriate place to receive care. All persons contacting the TNT line are triaged using evidence-based triage protocols developed by physicians. The person calling may take the advice of the nurse as to the most appropriate place to receive care, or the person may choose to receive care elsewhere. The TNT line serves all citizens of Midland County. Although this service has been in existence for a short time, initial data reveal satisfaction by patients, medical providers, and clinicians. In addition to the original intent of serving the county residents, the TNT is listed as a source by a competing hospital, and the TNT has received calls from as far away as Washington DC.

The use of TNT services in all communities should be considered in improving the appropriate use of EDs across the nation. Protecting this high-cost, resource-intensive service for appropriate usage is an obligation of any community-focused organization.

Hospital EDs are in crisis. The ED has become a linchpin of the health care safety net, with a high level of inappropriate users.[23,27] Significant barriers to obtaining access to primary care result in patients seeking nonurgent care in EDs.[19] One strategy is to increase the appropriate use of the ED, and effective TNT seems to achieve that outcome.

Leaders must recognize the performance of a department or process through collecting and analyzing key data in the problem-solving process. A review of the literature may give the leader ample evidence for implementing new or improved practices. Leaders who share the findings with stakeholders and gain support for change will show the best improvements.

REFERENCES

1. Bureau, U.S. Census.(n.d.). American fact finder. US. Census Bureau's. American Fact Finder. Available at: http://factfinder.census.gov/servlet/ACSSAFFFacts?_event=ChangeGeoContext&geo_id=05000US48329&_geoContext=&_street=&_county=Midland&_cityTown=Midland&_state=04000US48&_zip=&_lang=en&_sse=on&ActiveGeoDiv=&_useEV=&pctxt=fph&pgs1=010&_submenuId=factsheet_1&d. Accessed August 14, 2009.
2. Wilson L. Medical Director, Emergency Services at MMH (R.L. Dent, Interviewer). 2008, August.
3. Yoon P, Steiner I, Reinhardt G. Analysis of factors influencing length of stay in the emergency department. CJEM 2003;5(3):155–61.
4. Fortune T. Telephone triage: an Irish view. Accid Emerg Nurs 2001;9:152–6.
5. Fry M, Stainton C. An educational framework for triage nursing based on gatekeeping, timekeeping and decision-making processes. Accid Emerg Nurs 2005;13:214–9.
6. Funderburke P. Exploring best practice for triage. J Emerg Nurs 2008;34(2):180–2.
7. Light PA, Hupcey JE, Clark MB. Nursing telephone triage and its influence on parents' choice of care for febrile children. J Pediatr Nurs 2005;20(6):424–9.
8. Cariello FP. Computerized telephone nurse triage. An evaluation of service quality and cost. J Ambul Care Manage 2003;26(2):124–37.
9. Code Red Task Force. Code Red: the critical condition of health in Texas. Available at: http://coderedtexas.org/. 2008. Accessed January 31, 2009.
10. Cooke T, Watt D, Wertzler W, et al. Patient expectations of emergency department care: phase II—a cross-sectional survey. CJEM 2006;8(3):148–57.
11. Greenberg ME. Telephone nursing: evidence of client and organization benefits. Nurs Econ 2000;18(3):117–23.
12. Hagan L, Morin D, Lepine R. Evaluation of telenursing outcomes: satisfaction, self-care practices, and cost savings. Public Health Nurs 2000;17(4):305–13.
13. Keatinge D, Rawlings K. Outcomes of a nurse-led telephone triage services in Australia. Int J Nurs Pract 2005;11(1):5–12.
14. Dale J, Williams S, Foster T, et al. Safety of telephone consultations from 'non-serious' emergency ambulance service patients. Qual Saf Health Care 2004;13:363–73.

15. Emergency Nurses Association. Position statement telephone advice. Emergency Nurses Association, 2001. Available at: http://www.ena.org/about/position/pdfs/telephoneadvice.pdf. Accessed January 31, 2009.

16. Etter R, Ludwig R, Lersch R, et al. Early prognostic value of the medical emergency team calling criteria in patients admitted to intensive care from the emergency department. Crit Care Med 2008;36(3):775–81.

17. Larson-Dahn M. Tel-eNurse Practice: quality of care and patient outcomes. J Nurs Adm 2001;31(3):145–52.

18. Abad-Grau MM, Ierache J, Cervino C, et al. Evolution and challenges in the design of computational systems for triage assistance. J Biomed Inform 2008; 41(3):432–41.

19. Brim C. A descriptive analysis of the non-urgent use of emergency departments. Nurse Res 2008;15(3):72–88.

20. Lowe RA, Localio AR, Schwarz DF, et al. Association between primary care practice characteristics and emergency department use in a Medicaid Managed Care Organization. Med Care 2005;43(8):792–800.

21. Marklund B, Ström M, Mänson J, et al. Computer-supported telephone nurse triage: an evaluation of medical quality and costs. J Nurs Manag 2007;15(2): 180–7.

22. O'Connell JM, Towles W, Yin M, et al. Patient decision making: use of and adherence to telephone-based nurse triage recommendations. Med Decis Making 2002;22(4):309–17.

23. O'Rourke KM, Roddy M, King R, et al. Impact of a nursing triage. Line on the use of emergency department services in a military hospital. Mil Med 2003;168(12): 981–5.

24. Raper J, Davis BA, Scott L. Patient satisfaction with emergency department triage nursing care: a multicenter study. J Nurs Care Qual 1999;13(6):11–24.

25. Ruger JP, Lewis LM, Richter CJ. Identifying high-risk patients for triage and resource allocation in the ED. Am J Emerg Med 2007;25(7):794–8.

26. Wennike N, Williams E, Frost S, et al. Nurse-led triage of acute medical admissions: accurate and time-efficient. Br J Nurs 2007;16(13):824–7.

27. Wetta-Hall R, Ablah E, Dismuke S, et al. Emergency department use by people on low income. Emerg Nurse 2005;13(3):12–8.

Different Worlds: A Cultural Perspective on Nurse-Physician Communication

Carol A. Mannahan, EdD, RN, NEA-BC

KEYWORDS

• Culture • Collaboration • Nurse-physician communication

Every day, health care professionals attired in various uniforms traipse out onto the playing field. Since we don't practice together, we are never sure of just what the game plan is. We never know what our teammates are going to do next.

Some hog the ball. Others insist on running to opposing goals. No one seems to know the score. Watching doctors and nurses play, you'd hardly know we are on the same side.[1]

In the fast-paced world of modern health care, poor working relationships seem to be at the core of many patient safety issues. In fact, despite an abundance of data that points to the positive impact of physician-nurse collaboration on patient outcomes, most would agree with Chenevert's observation that physicians and nurses do not work well together. Specifically, ineffective nurse-physician communication has been linked to increased patient mortality, increased cost, longer lengths of stay, and rising error rates.[2,3] Other investigators have linked poor nurse-physician communication with physician and nurse job dissatisfaction and increases in nursing job stress.[4–6]

Current pressures in the health care system have moved nurse-physician communication from a long-standing concern to center stage. For example, an important element of a Magnet hospital is good working relationships between nurses and physicians.[7] The Institute of Medicine, the Joint Commission, and others have created standards demanding that the problem of poor nurse-physician communication be resolved. Indeed, a fresh approach to an old problem is needed. Because the worlds of medicine and nursing are at times referred to as "different cultures," a glimpse into what is known about culture and achieving cultural competence provides nursing leaders with new perspectives with which to improve relationships with physician colleagues.

University of Oklahoma College of Nursing, Oklahoma City, 3812 Mason Hills Drive, PO Box 3074, Edmond, OK 73083, USA
E-mail address: carol@mannahan.com

Nurs Clin N Am 45 (2010) 71–79
doi:10.1016/j.cnur.2009.10.005
0029-6465/10/$ – see front matter © 2010 Elsevier Inc. All rights reserved.

A CULTURAL PERSPECTIVE

For over 3 decades, health professionals have grappled with the need to deliver cultur-ally sensitive care to diverse patient populations. Experts agree that culture is a learned pattern of beliefs, customs, language, norms, and values that is held by a group of people. Extending beyond ethnicity, culture has come to mean a way of life that is accepted without thinking and is passed along by communication and imitation from one generation to the next. Further, scholars[8,9] agree that culture

- Develops over time and is responsive to its members
- Is learned and shared by members
- Is essential for survival and acceptance
- Is difficult to change.

Transcultural nursing models began to emerge less than 30 years ago because of the need to work with people from widely divergent backgrounds. Leininger's Culture Care Theory[10] defined transcultural nursing as a legitimate and formal area of study, research, and practice focused on culturally based care and values. Yet, most have difficulty "seeing beyond" their own culture and experiences. Leininger referred to "ethnocentrism" as the perception that one's own way is best when viewing the world. Although it is a natural behavior, Leininger pointed out that ethnocentrism is a major barrier to working effectively with diverse cultures. Although they frequently discuss physician issues with one another, nurses seldom venture outside of the nursing culture to resolve differences.

Further, recent literature related to cultural competence indicates that rather than approaching it as a set of stereotypical behaviors, it is more useful to seek understanding of the culture and its individual members. In his blockbuster book *The 7 Habits of Highly Effective People*, Covey[11] pointed out that it is more impor-tant to understand than to be understood when he discussed the fifth "habit," mutual understanding. He warned that giving advice before thoroughly listening to another person's concerns will likely result in the advice being rejected. Burke and colleagues[5] reported that nurses often express frustration that their concerns are not acknowledged, and that their recommendations are often rejected.

A CULTURAL COMPETENCE MODEL

Despite the widespread acknowledgment that nurses and physicians do function in different cultures, strategies for achieving cultural competence have not been applied to working relationships of these groups. Campinha-Bacote's model[12,13] has been empirically tested and applied in a variety of settings. A well-respected framework for guiding clinical practitioners, this model acknowledges the complexity of internal-ized culture and provides a structure for examining the worlds of nursing and medicine from a cultural perspective.

Several definitions support the application of cultural competence as a strategy for better understanding gaps in nurse-physician communication. For example, early work in this area saw cultural competence as a set of congruent behaviors, attitudes, and policies that come together among professionals and enable them to work effec-tively in cross-cultural situations. Pedersen's multicultural competence model[9] emphasized 3 components: awareness, knowledge, and skills. Denoba[14] defined cultural competence as simply the level of knowledge-based skills required to provide effective clinical care to patients from a particular ethnic or racial group; Betancourt and colleagues[15] defined it as a developmental process that evolves over an extended period. Campinha-Bacote's Model of Cultural Competence in Health Care Delivery[12,13] expanded the concept of cultural competence with the addition of the following 5 constructs:

- **Awareness**: self-examination of one's own cultural and professional background; recognition of own bias, prejudices, and assumptions about those who are different
- **Knowledge**: seeking and obtaining a sound educational foundation about the worldview of diverse groups
- **Cultural skill**: the ability to conduct a cultural assessment to collect relevant cultural data
- **Encounters**: direct engagement in cross-cultural interactions to modify existing beliefs about a cultural group
- **Desire**: intrinsic qualities of motivation & genuine caring of the health care provider to want to become culturally competent.

APPLICATION OF A MODEL

The Campinha-Bacote model works well in the nurse-physician cultural competence context. This model provides an excellent starting point for nursing leaders to design strategies to bridge cultural differences between nurses and physicians. Physicians and nurses are educated to work with culturally diverse patient populations. Integration of a cultural perspective to better understand the culture of physicians does not imply new knowledge—it merely requires a broader view of current practice expectations.

Guided by the "right questions" ("ASKED") proposed by Campinha-Bacote,[12,13] the following application of her model is suggested.

Awareness

Am I aware of my biases and prejudices towards other cultural groups?
The ability to identify, assess, and manage one's own emotions is often referred to as emotional intelligence. Goleman[16] popularized the idea that self-knowing is a prerequisite for emotional maturity, healthy relationships, and the capacity for empathy in his best-selling book *Emotional Intelligence: Why It Can Matter More Than IQ*. Goleman wrote that an accurate sense of self-mastery and the ability to withstand emotional storms has been praised as a virtue since Plato's time. Campinha-Bacote contended that it is a critical element of cultural competence.

An accurate self-assessment demands that nurses acknowledge personal biases they may hold toward physicians, especially when there is a point of disagreement. Self-assessment requires that nurses face the sense of powerlessness that they may have attributed to physicians and admit that they have allowed themselves to be victimized by the need for physician approval at the same time they are struggling to identify an independent role for nurses.

Self-assessment also requires nurses to consider personal factors that may affect relationships with physicians. For example, physicians consistently cite competence as essential to trust and respect.[17] In addition to educational level of Bachelor of Science in Nursing or greater, Schmalenberg and colleagues[17] reported that to physicians, nurse competence can be measured by national certification and how well they give report, particularly by phone in emergency situations. Kramer[18] concluded that competence in the performance of one's own role is a key factor in collaborative nurse-physician relationships.

Knowing the value of competence to physicians and some ways that they determine competence in nurses, nurses must consider what they are doing to stay current in their practice and to demonstrate their competence to others. Visible posting of nurse certifications and awards as well as integration of evidence-based practice strategies into their practice demonstrates an ongoing effort by nurses to deliver the best possible care. In contrast, the common practice of floating nurses between units to address staff shortages needs to be evaluated for its effect on competence. Nurses consistently report that floating puts them in situations where they are uncomfortable with their ability to function effectively.

In addition, gender differences have historically contributed to nurse-physician conflict. It was thought that as more women entered medicine, difference would be less of a factor. However, because men continue to dominate the ranks of established medical practitioners, it is likely that female physicians continue to be socialized to respond in ways similar to their male counterparts. In the study by Coeling and Wilcox,[19] physicians (male and female) focused primarily on the content aspect of the message and nurses placed more value on the relationship aspect of the message. Appropriate gender communication is an example of a social pattern that adds diversity and knowledge to the interaction and thus enhances collaboration.[20]

Finally, use of instruments such as the Myer-Briggs Type Indicator (MBTI) helps nurses to gain a better understanding of their preferred styles of interaction, temperament, learning styles, and problem solving. Such tools help individuals to understand themselves and their behaviors, recognize differences in others, and value different ways of approaching problems.

Skills

Do I have the skill to conduct a cultural assessment in a sensitive manner?

Cultural assessment is recognized as an effective strategy to gain insight into the norms, values, and beliefs of other cultures. Application of this strategy to the culture of physicians can assist nurses toward the greater understanding that Covey suggested.

A review of cultural assessment tools revealed several common elements that could be adapted to an assessment of the culture of physicians. These elements and examples of assessment items are presented in **Table 1** as a starting point for nursing leaders who choose to develop a tool to assess the culture of their physicians.

Knowledge

Am I knowledgeable about the world views of different cultural and ethnic groups?

Physicians historically have assumed a directive role in patient care, and nurses have functioned primarily to carry out their orders. Although both disciplines acknowledge the value of teamwork and collaboration, *interdisciplinary* teamwork and collaboration are not stressed in the education of either discipline. Because physicians typically see themselves as the dominant player in patient care, they are not likely to seek out nurses for collaboration. Casanova and colleagues[7] suggested that physicians sometimes view collaboration with nurses as undermining the physician's authoritarian role.

Benner[21] pointed out that that one's professional role is likely attained during professional education and early in practice. Fundamental differences in the education and practice of nurses and physicians exist. Nursing education is at the baccalaureate level or less. Medical education occurs at the graduate level, often with additional science degrees. Individuals can practice nursing with as little as 2 years' education post high school. On the other hand, physicians have 6 to 8 years of higher education. Physicians still perceive that nurses are "trained" and expect them to perform tasks. Although they express a desire for nurses to use critical thinking skills, they are often

Table 1 Physician cultural assessment	
Examples: Cultural Assessment Items	Examples: Physician Culture Assessment
Language and communication process	• How would you like for nurses to contact you when we are concerned about a patient? • Do you find S-BAR format to be a helpful way for us to update you about patients?
Values orientation	• What things are important to you regarding your relationship with nurses and the staff on this unit? • What specific nursing behaviors are the most helpful to you? The most frustrating?
Cultural health beliefs and practices	• For what types of patient issues do you want nurses to contact you immediately? • What things would you like to know about your patients when you make rounds on the unit?
Habits, customs, and beliefs	• Do you have any specific equipment or other preferences that would make your work on this unit easier? • What do you want us (nursing staff) to know about your practice and expectations?

Abbreviation: S-BAR, Situation-Background-Assessment-Recommendation.

surprised that nurses may have advanced degrees; many admit that they have no idea about nursing educational preparation at any level. Because of the wide range of nursing education, physicians are often confused about a nurse's level of knowledge and what they can expect from nurses.

Difference in both age and clinical experience between newly graduated nurses and new physicians adds to misunderstandings. Such differences are clear to see when considering the possibility of a 20-year-old associate degree new graduate working with a 33-year-old new cardiologist who has completed several years of residency. Although the average age of Associate Degree in Nursing nurses is typically older than 20, age differences do exist and the amount of clinical exposure between a new nurse and a new physician is quite different.

Along with differences in education, age, and clinical experiences, differences in approach to practice may lead to problems in nurse-physician working relationships. Despite changes in provider arrangements, physicians still approach their practices as self-employed entrepreneurs. Physicians determine who their patients are and the care patients will receive. Often caring for patients before hospitalization, physicians often continue care after discharge. Physicians often have patients on more than one unit or more than one hospital. An important factor in physician approach to practice is that individual physicians are solely accountable for the outcomes of their patients.

On the other hand, many nurses continue to be hospital employees. In addition to their responsibility for patient care, they are accountable to their employer, the institution. Nurses have no control over the patients admitted to their unit and typically have no contact with patients before or after the hospital stay. Although individual nurses are accountable for their actions, they have a chain of command through which they function. As a result, accountability for outcomes is a shared accountability between nurses, managers, and others within the institution.

Finally, Larsen[22] reported that the quality of the nurse-physician relationship was clearly of more concern to nurses than physicians. In a meta-analysis of studies pertaining to nurse-physician relationships over a 5-year period, 64% of the citations appeared in nursing journals; 29.5% were in medical journals. Also, although nurses and physicians both reported awareness of the importance of collaboration, nurses consistently rated the quality of the relationships lower than physicians.

Encounters

Do I seek out face-to-face and other types of interactions with individuals who are different from me?

Although ineffective communication is often cited as a problem, structures to improve communication between nurses and physicians are often lacking in daily practice. A good way to improve this problem is with introductions—physicians often want to know who is caring for their patients. New nurses should be introduced to unit physicians, and physicians appreciate it when any staff member greets them and updates them about their patients. Some physicians might find it helpful to see nurse names and photographs posted outside patient rooms.

Because they tend to have short parcels of time (unlike nurses for whom patient care is ongoing throughout a shift), physicians value concise and relevant information at a time when they are focused on a specific patient. Nurse-physician rounding meets communication needs for both disciplines. During rounds, nurses can update physicians about the patient's condition, clarify unclear orders, and participate in planning future care. On rounds, nurses can encourage patients to express their wishes clearly. Communication with family members is more effective if nurses are aware of physician plans. Effective communication during rounds can reduce the need to contact physicians at other times, which is disruptive to both nurses and physicians.

Strategies to coordinate rounds with multiple physicians and balance patient and unit needs can be worked out. For example, on one unit each nurse may choose to make rounds with each unit physician once per week. Another unit may assign nurses to make daily rounds with specific physicians based on teams or patient care assignments. Strategies may vary if the purpose of rounds is clear to physicians and nurses, and if nursing leaders value and support nurse-physician rounding.

By encouraging opportunities for nurses and physicians to interact away from the bedside, nursing leaders increase the chance for positive working relationships to develop between their staff and physicians. Examples of this include inviting physicians to speak at staff meetings and educational sessions, including them in unit functions, cosponsoring educational events, and attending physician meetings that address patient care and quality issues. Work with interdisciplinary groups such as institutional review boards and ethics committees are excellent ways to learn more about physician values and beliefs. Another strategy, expecting physicians and nurses to work together to address patient complaints with which they are involved, sends a clear message that nurses and physicians are a team with ultimate accountability to the patient.

As nurses seek additional professional interactions with physicians, the impact of appearance, demeanor, and even language and its effect on other cultures needs to be considered. Because these factors are often tied to first impressions, it is likely that they initially contribute to the degree of respect and trust that develops. For nurses seeking to cross the cultural divide between medicine and nursing, it is wise to approach physicians with confidence and to be sure that their appearance, demeanor, and language communicate professionalism that is worthy of respect and trust.

Table 2 Application of Lewin's model of change	
Lewin's Force-Field Model of Change	**Application of Model**
1. Unfreezing	Recognize physician relationship problems and reduce the forces that maintain the status quo • Provide opportunities for staff to express concerns about physician relationships • Post and discuss current research that links quality of physician-nurse relationships with patient outcomes • Encourage nurses who have healthy relationships with physicians to model their behavior to staff and nursing students
2. Moving	Develop goals and objectives to change the relationship; plan and implement strategies; promote new values, attitudes, and behaviors • Identify staff change-champions to work with peers to create a plan for better understanding of physician's culture • Adopt a cultural competency model to use as a guide • Include physicians and other stakeholders in the change process
3. Refreezing	Reinforce improved physician relationships; new behaviors, values, and attitudes are expected • Include physician relationships on staff meeting agendas • Join physicians on their rounds • Encourage attendance at interdisciplinary meetings • Include development of positive interdisciplinary relationships as part of the RN evaluation • Evaluate and revise relationship-building strategies regularly

Desire

Do I really "want to" become culturally competent?

The desire for "steady state" or keeping the status quo is powerful in individuals and organizations. For leaders who must initiate change and innovation to keep up with a rapidly changing health care system, resistance to change is a constant challenge. Integration of cultural competence in education and practice is an example of how slowly change occurs. Despite over 3 decades of research and knowledge about the impact of culture on health care, inclusion of this concept has only recently become common practice.

Evidence indicates that most nurses are not satisfied with their current relationship with physicians. Because nurses typically view problems in the relationship as originating with physicians, they may resist the idea of changing their behavior despite the awareness that changing oneself is far easier than changing another.

Numerous change theories, models, and frameworks have been promoted to guide individual and organizational change. Because of its simplicity and familiarity to many nurses, Lewin's Force-Field Model of Change[23] is an effective tool to guide reluctant nurses to a deeper understanding of physician culture. Application of this and other models helps leaders to plan consistent approaches to change that acknowledge organizational and personal impediments to the process. **Table 2** illustrates use of Lewin's 3-part model to guide changes in nurse interactions with physicians.

SUMMARY

In the effort to address cultural differences between nurses and physicians, one must remember that there are many shared values between the 2 cultures. As Campinha-

Bacote[12,13] pointed out, there is often more variation within a culture than between cultures. In health care, the variations may be more related to how one works toward goals rather than the goals themselves. For example, both nurses and physicians generally have the well-being of patients as their purpose and passion. Both are willing to work hard, and appreciate a pleasant work environment and colleagues whom they can respect for their compassion and competence. Both nurses and physicians know that communication is a crucial part of their roles and that neither can do alone all the work that needs to be done in health care. Most nurses and physicians understand that cross-cultural communication involves having respect for, tolerance of, and nonjudgmental attitudes toward people with different attitudes, behaviors, and values. Moreover, they know that stereotypes can be dangerous in matters of culture—they often result in negative self-fulfilling prophesies that create barriers to the understanding sought.

As nurses continue to seek better ways to build sound professional relationships with physician colleagues, one should remember that cross-cultural communication occurs when someone from one culture correctly understands a message sent by someone from another culture, and that the root of cultural competence begins with knowledge of the culture and sensitivity to the differences.

REFERENCES

1. Chenevert M. The pro-nurse handbook. St Louis (MO): Mosby; 1993. p. 9.
2. Baggs J, Schmitt M, Mishlin AI, et al. Association between nurse-physician collaboration and patient outcomes in three intensive care units. Crit Care Med 1999;27(9):1991–8.
3. Schmalenberg C, Kramer M, King C, et al. Excellence through evidence: securing collegial/collaborative nurse-physician relationships, part II. J Nurs Adm 2005;35(11):507–14.
4. Boyle D, Kochinda C. Enhancing collaborative communication of nurse and physician leadership in two intensive care units. J Nurs Adm 2004;34(2):60–70.
5. Burke M, Boal J, Mitchell R. Communicating for better care. Am J Nurs 2004; 104(12):40–7.
6. Cowan M, Shapiro M, Hays R, et al. The effect of a multidisciplinary hospitalist/ physician and advanced practice nurse collaboration on hospital costs. J Nurs Adm 2006;36(2):79–85.
7. Casanova J, Day K, Dorpat D, et al. Nurse-physician work relations and role expectations. J Nurs Adm 2007;37(2):68–70.
8. Campinha-Bacote J. The process of cultural competence in the Delivery of Healthcare Services: the journey continues. 5th edition. Cincinnati (OH): Transcultural C.A.R.E. Associates; 2007.
9. Pederson P. A handbook of developing multicultural awareness. Alexandria (VA): American Association for Counseling and Development; 1988.
10. Leininger M. What is transcultural nursing and culturally competent care? J Transcult Nurs 1999;13(3):189–92.
11. Covey S. The 7 habits of highly effective people. New York: Simon and Schuster; 1989.
12. Campinha-Bacote J. The process of cultural competence in the delivery of healthcare services: a model of care. J Transcult Nurs 2002;13(3):181–4.
13. Campinha-Bacote J. Cultural competence in psychiatric nursing: have you ASKED the right questions? J Am Psychiatr Nurses Assoc 2002;8(16):183–7.

14. Denoba D. MCHB/DSCSHCN guidance for competitive applications, maternal and child health improvement projects for children with special health care needs. Washington, DC: U.S. Department of Health and Human Services, Health Services and Resources Administration; 1993.
15. Betancourt J, Green A, Carrillo E. Cultural competence in health care: emerging frameworks and practical approaches. New York (NY): The Commonwealth Fund; 2002.
16. Goleman D. Emotional intelligence: why it can matter more than IQ. New York: Bantam Books; 1995.
17. Schmalenberg C, Kramer M, King C, et al. Excellence through evidence: securing collegial/collaborative nurse-physician relationships, part I. J Nurs Adm 2005;35(10):450–7.
18. Kramer M, Schmalenberg C. Development and evaluation of essentials of magnetism tool. J Nurs Adm 2004;34(7/8):1–14.
19. Coeling H, Wilcox J. Steps to collaboration. Nurs Adm Q 1994;18(4):44–55.
20. Gardner D. Ten lessons in collaboration. Online J Issues Nurs 2005;10(1).
21. Benner P. From novice to expert: excellence and power in clinical nursing practice. Menlo Park (CA): Addison-Wesley; 1984.
22. Larsen E. The impact of physician-nurse interaction on patient care. Holist Nurs Pract 1999;3(2):38–46.
23. Lewin K. Group and social change. In: Newcomb T, Hartley E, editors. Readings in social psychology. New York: Holt, Rhinehart, and Winston; 1947.

Evidence-Based Staffing and "Communityship" as the Key to Success

Karlene Kerfoot, PhD, RN, NEA-BC, FAAN[a],*, Kathy Douglas, MHA, RN[b]

KEYWORDS

- Evidence-based staffing • Communityship • Lean
- Zero-defect health care

Staffing can spell success or failure for the nurse leader at either the executive level or the frontline level. Effective staffing creates excellence in quality outcomes, nurse satisfaction, retention and safety, patient loyalty, and reputation of the organization. Financially, effective staffing affects the bottom line, and now that pay for performance, decreased tolerance for errors, and poor clinical outcomes are part of the reimbursement picture, interest in staffing is escalating. New research and evidence about the relationship of effective staffing to patient, nurse, and organizational outcomes are also available. Previously, leaders intuitively knew that staffing effectiveness was tied to patient outcomes, but it was difficult to quantify because the research was not available. That is no longer the case. Good evidence is available describing the relationship of evidence-based practice and the outcomes of staffing. The challenge is how to move from opinion-based staffing models to rapidly embedding evidence-based models that improve the quality of care available to patients.

APPLYING EVIDENCE-BASED DATA TO STAFFING

Although the use of evidence to drive quality is widely understood and used in clinical practice, this is less true when applying evidence to staffing practices. The importance of analyzing the needs of the patient and understanding the competencies of staff and the call to routinely evaluate staffing effectiveness on patients' outcomes have been highlighted in the literature.[1–3] The white paper, *Excellence and Evidence in Staffing; Essential Links to Staffing Solutions for Health care*,[4] is the product of a summit on evidence-based staffing at which input from more than 50 health care leaders from community and academic hospitals, academia, professional nursing organizations,

[a] Aurora Health Care, 3000 West Montana, Milwaukee, WI 53234, USA
[b] Institute for Staffing Excellence & Innovation, 535 Grow Drive, Sedona, AZ 86336, USA
* Corresponding author.
E-mail address: karlene.kerfoot@aurura.org (K. Kerfoot).

Nurs Clin N Am 45 (2010) 81–87
doi:10.1016/j.cnur.2009.10.006   nursing.theclinics.com
0029-6465/10/$ – see front matter © 2010 Published by Elsevier Inc.

and industry was generated. This report provides a review of the literature and maps the research to substantiate 10 best practice recommendations. At the center of this work is a model for evidence-based staffing that demonstrates the importance of applying the available evidence to staffing by making evidence/science the foundation of the model. The paper also points out the importance of understanding staffing and its broad implications for the operational and financial performance of a health care organization. We now have significant evidence-based studies about staffing to base much of our practice on evidence. Clark[5] notes that we now have the evidence to justify investments in nurse staffing and high-quality practice environments. Our challenge is to infuse this information throughout the organization so that integrated evidence-based decisions are made in every part of the organization that affects patient care.

EVIDENCE-BASED STAFFING AS AN INTEGRATED COLLABORATIVE PROCESS AND "COMMUNITYSHIP"

Historically the work of staffing has been considered the accountability of the Chief Nursing Officer (CNO) or designee. However, effective staffing is influenced by a great number of people and processes in the organization that are outside the direct responsibilities of the CNO. Malloch and Porter O'Grady[6] describe how we are leaving the industrial age and moving into an age in which it is clearly recognized that the integration of the parts into the whole is necessary for success and in which the interdependence of parts is clearly seen and recognized. The CNO then has to see the role from this perspective and manage the interconnections between people and processes. These authors also note that the old world order was focused on the processes, actions, work, tasks, functions, and jobs. In the present and evolving world, outcomes, results, and sustainable accomplishments have replaced the process-oriented industrial age thinking. The nurse leader cannot achieve effective staffing without the ability to manage these issues with the teams of people inside and outside nursing who can achieve the desired outcomes. Freshman and colleagues[7] note that the publication by the Committee on Quality of Health Care in America, Institute of Medicine,[8] described health care quality as suffering from the inability to work collaboratively across disciplines. Uncoordinated, sequential action that focuses on efficiency within silos instead of collaboration across boundaries has led to a system that is unsafe and uncoordinated. Staffing is a primary example of this state of health care. We cannot be effective without seeing staffing as an integrated, system-wide process and having discussions about evidence, quality, efficiency, and nursing care, independent of others in the organization.

Mintzberg[9] uses the term "communityship" to describe the style of leadership needed today. Mintzberg describes what he calls the harmful and pervasive leadership style we have been experiencing of leaders who sit in offices and announce the goals they want others to attain. They do not move out of their office and on to patient care areas to help people achieve these goals. The leader as isolated individualist must be morphed into a leader who is personally engaged and believes in distributed management. Mintzburg[9](p141) uses the terms "just enough leadership" and "communityship" to describe an alternative to the top-down centralized bureaucratic style of leadership. Communityship is an excellent concept to describe the work that is necessary to create effective staffing outcomes.

From Mintzberg's point of view, community is about "…caring about our work, our colleagues, and our place in the world, geographic and otherwise and in turn being inspired by this caring." He uses the term communityship as the alternate to the ndividualistic leadership model of the past. Companies such as Toyota and Pixar are examples of this style of leadership. An organization, according to Mintzberg, knows that it has arrived when its members reach out in socially responsible and mutually beneficial ways to each other.

Effective staffing takes a community. It requires that people reach out to each other over and through departmental firewalls to care for each other, for each other's work, and for the ultimate safety of patients and staff. When departments, such as finance, support departments, unions, pharmacy, and the nursing organization, can work across departmental lines to share the vision and execute evidence-based effective staffing, excellent outcomes can be achieved. The challenge is to measure outcomes by what happens to the patient, not by isolated department-specific numbers that include only compliance to budgeted numbers. The needed measure is the activities that have improved or worsened, based on the outcome of what the patient expects— zero-defect health care.

Staffing is an interactive system influenced by many people throughout the organization. Holds in the emergency department because of inadequate staffing in the intensive care units, lack of teamwork, staff turnover, unit turbulence, new physicians, inadequately stocked supplies, cumbersome computer systems, and unilateral decisions made in pharmacy, finance, or medical records are all examples of issues that affect staffing and the ability to achieve superior outcomes for patients. Effective evidence-based staffing is the result of interactive processes that cross many boundaries.

Moving an organization to an evidence-based model for staffing and for achieving the outcomes designated by the patient requires the integration of leaders and staff, a strong understanding of all of the interrelated forces at play, and a culture of collaboration and inclusion.[4] The importance of the proactive leadership of nursing in this situation cannot be overstated. Moving staffing into a key strategic initiative, that of building communityship around staffing, takes vision and the ability to effectively translate that vision into terms that can be understood and embraced by everyone, from the executive team and the finance and support departments to the nurse delivering bedside care and the patient.

EXAMPLES OF COMMUNITYSHIP IN STAFFING

There are many leaders who implement staffing programs grounded in the best practices for excellence and use an evidence-based model. Their experience can provide guideposts for those seeking to convert to an evidence-based approach to staffing. Haley and Thering[10] spoke about their transition to an evidence-based approach to staffing excellence as one that could not have been accomplished without the close working relationship that was developed between nursing and finance. They describe a healthy relationship with finance as one demonstrated by shared responsibility for financial outcomes of staffing practices. To achieve this relationship required spending time together and learning about each other's areas. It also required enabling the staffing decision makers and ensuring that they were knowledgeable about clinical, operational, and financial implications of staffing decisions. Bedside nurses also played a key role by becoming active participants in the staffing process. This process is highlighted as essential in the Best Practices defined in Excellence and Evidence in Staffing.[4]

This position of collaboration was also emphasized by Valentine and Doyle.[11] In a separate presentation about their journey to excellence in staffing, Doug Hughes, Director of Nursing, Paoli Hospital, pointed out the difference between quick fixes, such as offering bonuses, and an investment in solutions that bring about sustainable change as the core of an excellence in staffing program.

Jeff Turner[12] described an example of Moore County Hospital's Chief Executive Officer (CEO), who has led, in partnership with nursing and others, a redesign of staffing practices that examines the underlying causes as the key to successful financial outcomes related to staffing. This CEO demonstrated a deep understanding of all of the forces at play related to staffing and the kind of informed leadership that can successfully lead the change to an evidence-based approach to staffing. Turner also points out the importance of the entire team as necessary to achieving the success that the Moore County Hospital is enjoying.

Suellyn Ellerbe,[13] an early innovator in evidence-based staffing programs, has led the change that empowered evidence-based staffing at many organizations. Citing collaboration, education, organizational awareness, and increased sense of responsibility across all stakeholders as keys to success, she has been able to achieve remarkable financial and operational outcomes, saving her organizations millions of dollars.

Block[14] notes that our organizations are plagued with fragmentation, disconnection, and detachment that make it virtually impossible for them to reach their full potential. For Block, leadership is conversation. Block also notes that we are most effective when we focus on others' gifts and not deficiencies. His asset-based conversations focus on possibilities among people and eliminate fragmentation. These examples demonstrate how leaders have taken the responsibility to have conversations with various other people in the organization to effectively eliminate fragmentation and change outcomes for patients.

INTEGRATED DECISION MAKING AND EFFECTIVE EVIDENCE-BASED NURSING ACROSS BOUNDARIES

When key stakeholders in the organization become familiar with evaluating decisions based on evidence and the effect on others in the health care process and the evidence, we will achieve a new level of integrated decision making that will create better outcomes. For example, decisions about information technology, clinical documentation, pharmacy processes, or renovation can positively or negatively affect effective staffing. When people who are not familiar with the staffing evidence make isolated decisions that radically affect nurse staffing, the organization is headed for a collision that produces poor patient outcomes and high costs. It will be impossible to reach staffing goals for efficiency and quality when decisions in another part of the organization can negatively affect the front line. A classic example is a process improvement effort in one department that decreases the workload and staff in that department but shifts the workload to the staff nurse without increasing nurse staffing. Just a few decisions like this in an organization will reduce the nurse's direct time at the bedside and will predictably, according to available evidence, create unwanted patient care outcomes, such as pressure ulcers or falls.

Unfortunately, it has been an all too common practice to reduce staff without taking their work out of the system. Processes such as applying Lean to hospitals[15] will provide the processes needed to make changes rather than relying on opinion-based productivity improvement initiatives that do not really improve productivity and quality in the long run. Lean methodologies have been used in hospitals effectively to reduce waste, which is defined as any problem that interferes with people doing their work effectively or any activity that does not provide value for the customer, who is defined as the nurse in some situations and the patient in others. Examples of reducing waste and saving nursing time are projects that have reduced the time nurses devote to hunting and gathering when supplies are not readily available because of stock-outs or when equipment are not available for immediate use, centralized rather than decentralized supplies that result in additional travel time for nurses, inefficient pharmacy procedures that result in endless phone calls and long patient waits, and nonnursing tasks delegated to nurses. Inefficient processes within nursing also create staffing issues for other departments. For example, an inefficient system of ordering missed medications from the pharmacy can result in the order being placed several times if the system cannot inform the nurse or pharmacist that the order has already been placed, and extra doses arrive on the unit. Hoarding of supplies and equipment by nurses, who because of their experience do not trust the supply system, results in incredible waste. When staffing reductions are made without looking at the root cause of inefficiencies across all systems and departments, then the decision only makes the inefficiencies worse. Lean technologies have much to teach everyone about intelligent redesign of processes.

The sole responsibility for staffing does not reside in the nursing department. Effective staffing is the result of integrated process improvement and decision making that creates synergy across boundaries and transparency across departmental borders.

COMMONALITIES OF SUCCESSFUL PROGRAMS

Reviewing these and many other examples surfaces some commonalities that can be helpful in supporting a move to an evidence-based approach to staffing.

- Involvement of stakeholder groups from all over the organization, including patients
- Strong understanding of interrelated forces
- Strong commitment to address underlying cause
- Education of all decision makers to a level of competency, not just those in nursing
- Shared responsibility for financial, operational, and clinical outcomes that create a feeling of integration and communityship.

Designing a program that embraces evidence-based staffing requires a strong understanding of the nurse staffing process and all of the complex interactive forces at play. Without a holistic, communityship view, there is risk in fixing something in one place only to find an unexpected consequence surface somewhere else in the system. Collaboration and participation across all stakeholder groups will lay the foundation for success and contribute to understanding the whole picture. It is the kind of collaboration that gives rise to new concepts like communityship. This thinking is fundamental to Magnet concepts. This new thinking becomes essential for realizing the operational, cultural, and financial outcomes necessary for achieving excellence in staffing. Investing in an environment in which participation and collaboration are embraced creates distributed ownership and accountability, which is a key success factor.

When there is a common understanding of the value that can be realized from taking an evidence-based and communityship approach to staffing, cooperation and innovation can thrive. Nurse executives must take an active role in promoting the understanding and value of evidence-based, communityship staffing within the executive team while also setting forth a vision for nursing. Nurse managers play a pivotal role in a successful staffing program, and investments in their understanding of not only the operational and clinical side of staffing but also the business side will yield high returns. Nurse managers who also embrace a communityship approach to leadership will find it easier to motivate their staff, promoting participation and initiating best practices, particularly those that promote successful working across departments.

The underpinning of success is awareness promoted through education and the underlying belief that when people understand something they will make the best decisions. Nursing needs to learn the language of the finance department and of other departments, and these same nonnursing groups need to learn more about direct care delivery. When staffing decisions are made, they should be made with a full understanding of the downstream implications of those decisions. Whether it is a budget discussion or solving a staffing problem on a given shift, all these decisions add up to affect patients, the workforce, and the organization in which care is delivered. In situations in which excellence in staffing thrives as an organizational value, accountability for outcomes is shared among leadership, management, and staff across departments. All areas have the understanding and motivation to support informed decision making for their particular aspect of the staffing world and the knowledge of potential implications of that decision on the rest of the staffing continuum.

INCLUDING THE PATIENT IN COMMUNITYSHIP: MOVING FROM NUMBER-CENTRIC STAFFING TO PATIENT-CENTRIC STAFFING OUTCOMES

Historically, staffing revolved around numbers such as hours per patient day or ratios, and the outcomes were to determine the numbers and to meet these numbers. We are now in the middle of a transformation where we are not judged on our process or our numbers. Instead, we are judged on the outcomes, as measured by patient outcomes such as pressure ulcers and falls. The challenge is to switch our thinking to measuring staffing effectiveness not by how well the numbers were met, but how the numbers influenced the creation of a defect-free health care system in which there are no pressure ulcers and no falls with injuries. Numbers alone will not reach this goal. A serious cross-departmental evaluation of the waste that is inherent in the process of delivering care to patients is what is needed. Eliminating the waste that takes staff time and does not contribute to excellence in outcomes is absolutely necessary. We cannot be effective unless we actively and continually apply methods such as those discussed by Graban[15] to improve processes and eliminate the waste that negates efficient and effective processes at the bedside. Cross-boundary interactions to constantly improve these processes must be embedded in the organization. Isolated department-only evaluation of staffing without assessing the downstream outcomes will not work.

Galbraith[16] tells us that there are 3 levels of customer-centric organizations, light level, medium level, and high level. On the trajectory to reach the high level, he notes that there are customer-facing structures close to the top that have the power to be a strong voice of the customer. These customer-facing processes are empowered to help shape the company's process and outcomes around what the customer wants, not what the company wants to sell. Health care has been challenged to seriously become patient-centered and to give up its departmental, profession-centered, inward-looking way of delivering health care. This approach is a critical change that we need to make in the way we view effective staffing. The customer has a right to and is demanding defect-free health care. With pay for performance, hospitals will not be paid for defects, and with public reporting of nurse-sensitive outcomes, patient satisfaction, and other outcomes, the defects become clear. Customers are giving us a clear message that the days of producing what we want without looking at what the customer is demanding for are over. We must move as soon as possible into the communityship of effective staffing that includes the patient to achieve that outcome.

SUMMARY

Embracing a leadership style that is inclusive and that leverages the ideas and input at all levels of an organization is the foundation of building an approach to staffing that maximizes outcomes for patients, the workforce, and the organizations in which care is delivered. By engaging everyone involved and inviting participation, a structure of shared understanding is created, providing an environment that is positioned to achieve optimal results. Communityship offers a model for approaching leadership that is aligned with leveraging talent across an organization and developing a culture prepared to face the complex challenges of staffing and achieving new levels of performance that an evidence-based approach to staffing excellence can offer. We are challenged to create a zero-defect health care system. We can do this only by becoming patient-centric, embedding effective evidence-based staffing programs, and developing communityship as the method to get us there.

REFERENCES

1. American Association of Critical Care Nurses. AACN standards for establishing and sustaining healthy work environments. Aliso Viejo (CA): AACN; 2005.
2. American Nurses Association. Principles for nurse staffing. Washington, DC: American Nurses Association; 1999.
3. American Organization of Nurse Executives. Policy statement on staffing ratios. Washington, DC: The American Organization of Nurse Executives; 2003.
4. Douglas K. Excellence and evidence in staffing. 2008. Available at: http://www. globalnursingnetwork.org. Accessed July 15, 2009.
5. Clark S. Making the business case for nursing: justifying investments in nurse staffing and high quality practice environments. Nurs Leadersh 2007;5(4):34–8.
6. Malloch K, Porter O'Grady T. Evidence-based practice in nursing and health care. New York: Jones & Bartlett; 2006.
7. Freshman B, Rubino L, Chassiakos YR. Collaboration across the disciplines in health care. New York: Jones & Bartlett; 2009.
8. Committee on Quality of Health Care in America, Institute of Medicine. Crossing the quality chasm: a new health system for the 21st century. New York: National Academies Press; 2001.
9. Mintzberg H. Rebuilding companies as communities. Harv Bus Rev 2009;87(7/8): 140–3.
10. Haley S, Theron DM. Nursing/finance collaboration more than just staffing; a vehicle for controlled change. IdeaConnect Webcast 2009.
11. Valentine N, Doyle J. Partnering with nursing to achieve cost effective staffing ANI. In: Healthcare Finance Conference. 2007.
12. Turner J. Staffing redesign drives financial performance: CEO and innovative team partner for success. IdeaConnect Webcast 2009.
13. Ellerbe S. Video interview. 2008. Available at: http://www.Ideaconnect2.com. Accessed July 15, 2009.
14. Block P. Community: the structure of belonging. New York: Berrett-Koehler; 2009.
15. Graban M. Lean hospitals improving quality, patient safety, and employee satisfaction. New York: Productivity Press; 2009.
16. Galbraith J. Designing the customer-centric organization. New York: Jossey-Bass; 2005.

Index

Note: Page numbers of article titles are in **boldface** type.

A

Accessibility, transformational leadership and application of Magnet's new empiric outcomes, 57–63

Advocacy, transformational leadership and application of Magnet's new empiric outcomes, 51–57

American Association of Nurse Executives (AONE), nurse executive competencies, 12

B

Behaviors, operational, conceptual framework for contemporary nurse executive practice, **33–38**
    new context for, 34
    new imperative for, 33–34
    one dozen cautions, 34–38

C

Camphina-Bacote model, cultural competence model for nurse-physician communication, **71–79**

Change, Lewin's model of, 77

Chief nursing officer (CNO), turnover, **11–31**
    analysis of literature on, 15–31
    impact of, 12
    unique role and perspective of, 12

Coaching, as an effective leadership intervention, **39–48**
    case study, 44–47
    literature review, 39–44

Collaboration, cultural competence model for nurse-physician communication, **71–79**

Communication, nurse-physician, cultural perspective on, **71–79**
    cultural competence model for, 72–77
    transformational leadership and application of Magnet's new empiric outcomes, 57–63

Communityship, evidence-based staffing and, as keys to success, **81–87**
    applying evidence-based data to, 81–82
    as an integrated collaborative process, 82–83
    commonalities of successful programs, 85–86
    examples of, 83–84
    including the patient in, 86
    integrated decision making and effective nursing across boundaries, 84–85

Competencies, for coaching as an effective leadership intervention, **39–48**
    for nurse executives, 11–12
    individual, for innovation leadership, 4–9

Nurs Clin N Am 45 (2010) 89–93
doi:10.1016/S0029-6465(10)00010-1
0029-6465/10/$ – see front matter © 2010 Elsevier Inc. All rights reserved.

nursing.theclinics.com

Moving?

Make sure your subscription moves with you!

To notify us of your new address, find your **Clinics Account Number** (located on your mailing label above your name), and contact customer service at:

Email: journalscustomerservice-usa@elsevier.com

800-654-2452 (subscribers in the U.S. & Canada)
314-447-8871 (subscribers outside of the U.S. & Canada)

Fax number: 314-447-8029

Elsevier Health Sciences Division
Subscription Customer Service
3251 Riverport Lane
Maryland Heights, MO 63043

*To ensure uninterrupted delivery of your subscription, please notify us at least 4 weeks in advance of move.

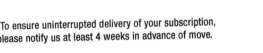

Printed and bound by CPI Group (UK) Ltd, Croydon, CR0 4YY
03/10/2024
01040445-0010